Online Health Forums and Services: Benefits, Risks and Perspectives

Authored by

Rita Mano

Department of Human Services,
University of Haifa,
Haifa, 3498838,
Israel

Online Health Forums and Services: Benefits, Risks and Perspectives

Author: Rita Mano

ISBN (Online): 978-981-14-9965-4

ISBN (Print): 978-981-14-9963-0

ISBN (Paperback): 978-981-14-9964-7

need for a court order if at any point you breach any terms of this License Agreement. In no event will any delay or failure by Bentham Science Publishers in enforcing your compliance with this License Agreement constitute a waiver of any of its rights.

3. You acknowledge that you have read this License Agreement, and agree to be bound by its terms and conditions. To the extent that any other terms and conditions presented on any website of Bentham Science Publishers conflict with, or are inconsistent with, the terms and conditions set out in this License Agreement, you acknowledge that the terms and conditions set out in this License Agreement shall prevail.

Bentham Science Publishers Pte. Ltd.
80 Robinson Road #02-00
Singapore 068898
Singapore
Email: subscriptions@benthamscience.net

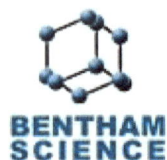

BENTHAM SCIENCE

CONTENTS

CONTENTS

PREFACE

A turning point to better health care includes the introduction of the Internet as a media source. Online access to health information and communication about health is associated with improved knowledge about health issues. Individuals in the past obtained information mainly through health professionals, their friends and families. They are now turning to virtual sources of information and social media to gather health information. They do so for a variety of reasons, including identifying symptoms of a health ailment and self-diagnosis, collecting knowledge on available treatment strategies and their effectiveness, evaluating the costs involved, and finding coping strategies for better self-management.

Individuals are becoming more aware and interested in adopting health changes in dietary and wellbeing routines. 61% of U.S. adults look online for health information, and the number of people using the Internet has almost tripled between 2011 and 2018, and more than 50% of users today look for online health information (Seth & Grant Harrington, 2018). Another recent survey indicates that 65% of online adults in the United States, or half of all US adults, use social media, with Facebook and Twitter being the most widely used (Madden & Zickuhr, 2017). Each minute, 695 000 Facebook statuses are updated, and 98,000 tweets are sent (Teiman, 2019). The use of online social media and online health forums for information seeking is especially noted when individuals face a serious health issue (Pew Research Center, 2013). "Dr. Google" has indeed become a favorite choice when seeking information from a virtual health center and was soon followed by the increase in the use of networking sites (Rosenberg *et al.*, 2017).

Following the rise of internet use, the phenomenon of digital health, including electronic health and mobile health, has risen as well. Using the web to access information and communication with peers can help individuals fulfill unmet informational needs and prepare them to consider changes in health habits. This is more likely for individuals who perceive the need for changing unhealthy habits to improve their health status when exposed to online information. In that sense, exposure to online health information through browsing and online communication might increase the likelihood of making a change in health habits empowering individuals to take responsibility for their health status (Lustria *et al.*, 2011; Pena-Purcell, 2008; Mano, 2018).

The health empowerment process involves the understanding that some means are better facilitators towards the desired health end. When individuals recognize their right to express aspirations and are able to define them as an outcome, they develop a critical "consciousness" of the existing situation. This consciousness increases their sense of self-efficacy (Bandura, 1997) and contributes to a healthy lifestyle throughout an individual's life span. The health empowerment process is possible by introducing, adjusting, and developing services that are easily accessed, regardless of lack of technical skills and basic health literacy (Mesch *et al.*, 2012; Mano, 2016; 2019) and is expanding among different social groups (Kummervold *et al.*, 2008; Wessels, 2013) shaped by individuals' health expectations and health attitudes. While technology plays a central role in health empowerment, knowledge alone cannot guarantee the adoption of healthy behaviors (Iverson *et al.*,2008; Shim *et al.*, 2006; Eisenberg & Berkowitz, 2009). Neither the access nor the use of the Internet is similar for all individuals in all social groups (Mano, 2017; 2019; Rosenberg *et al.*, 2020). As a result, health institutions and policy-makers encourage the development of services and programs that enable individuals to endorse the health empowerment process and assume responsibility for their own health needs, diagnosis, and treatment.

eHealth and mHealth technologies have enormous potential advancing health information exchange and improving healthcare access and public as well as personalized medicine (Bashshur and Shannon 2009; Wentzer and Bygholm 2013). The World Health Organization (WHO) and the International Telecommunication Union (ITU) defined the term "eHealth" as the field "concerned with improving the flow of information, through electronic means, to support the delivery of health services and the management of health systems" (p.1, World Health Organization, 2012c). A new definition shows that the World Health Organization (WHO; 2016) has defined Electronic Health (eHealth) as: "the cost-effective and secure use of information and communications technologies in support of health and health-related fields, including healthcare services, health surveillance, health literature, health education, knowledge, and research." WHO defined *Mobile Health (mHealth)* as: "mobile computing, medical sensor, and communications technologies for health care" (WHO, 2009). mHealth is also defined as the use of portable devices to deliver medical and public health services and is a subset of eHealth (Betjeman *et al.*, 2013; Wittet, 2012). Both phenomena are related to the commitment of individuals and health care providers to enhance healthcare and health management practices and form the basis of the health empowerment phenomenon which became a major theme in health-oriented western societies (Sillence *et al.*, 2007; Andreassen, *et al.*, 2007) often considered as the "holy grail of health promotion" (Rissel, 1994).

Health consumers arriving at the health provider with the information they found on the web, with a preconceived idea about their diagnosis, want to actively participate in therapeutic decisions relying on misleading or misinterpreted health information. Health institutions and health policy-makers prompt individuals to claim more responsibility, and they have eagerly employed technology to provide more effective and efficient services in order to handle health budgets in order to successfully combine between effective and efficient administration of virtual health devices (Aceijas, 2011; Mattke *et al.*, 2012; Balatsoukas *et al.*, 2015). These systems play a critical part in unifying communications, allowing people to access, process, store, and transmit data through fully integrated audiovisual, data communications, and electronic systems (Henriquez-Camacho *et al.*,2014). This means that the potential of social media to reach a large segment of the younger as well as the adult population searching for online insights to their health concerns. These systems seek to minimize digital divide effects and increase health literacy (Wessels, 2013) by introducing macro level systems based on online Information and communication technology (ICT).

At the same time, the empowered "Information control" process challenges the institutional health care provider into equality-based roles with patients. These challenges first and foremost included the outcomes of the shift in the "Information control" process from the authority of the institutional healthcare provider into the power of the informed individuals facing situations hardships in health. The empowered "Information control" process challenges the institutional health care provider into equality like roles with patients. In this process questions about differences in health attitudes and health behavior rise because knowledge alone cannot guarantee the adoption of healthy behaviors (Iverson *et al.*, 2008; Shim *et al.*, 2006; Eisenberg & Berkowitz, 2009).

Moreover, despite major investment in the development and introduction of advanced digital health services and programs, also seeking to reduce costs, health literacy is still low and access to online health services limited increasing doubts about the level of equality among socio economic groups. Even today the Internet is not accessible or used with similar levels of knowledge and skills in particular among the disadvantaged who need it most (Mattke *et al.*, 2012; Baran & Davis, 2009; Eisenberg & Berkowitz, 2009; Aceijas, 2011; Mano, 2016). Disadvantaged groups in terms of technology skills and/or access to online health information and services may ignore health issues, they do not ask for help and support, and have little motivation to deal with prevention of illness. The phenomenon of first and second-level effects of the digital divide is therefore discussed more often because they can affect health management and perhaps even life expectancy (Renahy *et al.*, 2008; Lorence *et al.*, 2006; Mesch *et al.* 2012; Rosenberg *et al.*, 2019). They terms describe lower investment in improved health whether or not they access online health services and the existence of mistrust (Gibbons, 2008; Mesch *et al.*,2012; Rosenberg *et al.*, 2019). As a result, health empowerment and successful self-management practices among those who need it most - the elderly, those located in remote geographic areas, and/or facing chronic illness and disabilities maybe missed (Hadwich *et al.*, 2006; Eisenberg & Berkowitz, 2009; Aceijas, 2011; Mano, 2016). This is why it is important to consider the sources of individual level variations in the health empowerment process including health attitudes, differences between health behaviors, trust and technology skills (Mano, 2019). The gap between the willingness and actual behavior to adopt digital services have profound impact for different sectors and they may affect decision making and allocation of resources to the online tools used by institutional health providers that manifest in the delivery of health services and health programs.

The purpose of this book is to provide the theoretical and empirical background to instigate an interdisciplinary perspective to issues of digital health in the 21st century.

In order to so, we discuss the factors associated with the use of online sources of health. The fundamental assumptions of this book refer to three dimensions of use of online forums for health purpose: first, at the micro level health attitudes and behaviors reflect a wide range of personal differences in terms of socioeconomic characteristics, technology skills, and preferences. Second, we refer to the quality of these sources of information regarding their suitability and accuracy is limited raising concerns about its usefulness to patients (Manchaiah *et al.*, 2020) raising doubts about the effectiveness of the health empowerment process. Third, we will discuss how variations at the individual level affect both the access and extent of use of virtual sources of health information and health services. Finally, we will present the basic problems associated with the use of virtual sources of health information and services at the level of institutional health practices and the association between the micro-level use of the Internet for health purposes and macro level challenges in the promotion of virtual sources of health products and health services.

We seek to present a comprehensive perspective that link between the aspects of the micro-level use of the Internet for health purposes (accessing health related websites, participation in health forums, bulletin boards and health related social networking sites) and the macro level practices of digital health that promote health empowerment. We also seek to identify the social and health characteristics of the different groups of patients and estimate to what extent individuals in need of health and medical information (chronic illness) are taking advantage of the availability of information and communication platforms to improve their health or are being left behind. More specifically, we intend to seek the differences in health outcomes - access to quantity and quality of health information, involvement in decision making empowerment in health behavior and health changes. In doing so, we refer to the following aspects of health:

1. access to online health information
2. use of online health services
3. social media and participation online health forums
4. mobile health applications and health risks
5. lifestyle health behaviors
6. self-management of health

7. digital divides in health
8. health systems

Due to its interdisciplinary nature, this book is a valuable source of empirical evidence information and theoretical contribution for an academic audience including students and researchers- as well as for public health practice institutions and policy makers. This is also a valuable source of those working in the field of health for the general public who have become very much health-aware these recent years since the internet has allowed for a great number of individuals a quick and immediate access to health information. Finally, the book enables a wide-audience friendly approach to issues of health to be used in connection with teaching, training and consulting activity in digital health. As the importance of particular and general concerns increases among the public, affecting current health policies, so does the importance of understanding the patterns of access and use of online platforms. After all, knowledge and information alone cannot guarantee the adoption of healthy behaviors (Iverson *et al.*, 2008; Eisenberg & Berkowitz, 2009).

CONSENT FOR PUBLICATION

Not applicable

CONFLICT OF INTEREST

The authors declare no conflict of interest, financial or otherwise.

ACKNOWLEDGEMENTS

Declared none.

Rita Mano
Department of Human Services
University of Haifa
Haifa, 3498838
Israel

CHAPTER 1

Theories

The internet is an integral part of the lives of millions of people around the world. It has brought about changes in individuals' social, political, and economic practices (Srinivasan & Fish, 2017) and has promoted the introduction of new forms of thinking and new assumptions about the central role of digital communications and information in everyday life. Online health searches, online health services and social media on health websites, blogs, and portals are all easily accessed (Li *et al.* 2015; Lin *et al.* 2016). These new trends have intrigued academic researchers, who aspire to find new paradigms to explain these trends. Theories and paradigms play a paramount role in understanding issues related to health. All theories, both old and new, seek to determine how society, individuals, and health behaviors and outcomes are related. Often the choice of a particular theory or paradigm can lead to different and sometimes contradictory hypotheses, resulting in different outcomes for similar data. Here, we provide a glimpse into the prominent theories of health and technology.

SOCIOLOGICAL THEORIES OF HEALTH AND TECHNOLOGY

Studies addressing issues of health in sociology are divided into two principal groups: sociology in medicine and sociology of medicine (Bradby *et al.*, 2017). The first group focuses on the role of sociologists in providing guidelines to various sponsors in health-related fields, among them government agencies, foundations, hospitals, or medical schools. They do this by developing health surveys that address topics related to health care, including access to care, use of services, health status determinants, and more (Higgs & Gilleard, 2015). The second group of studies focuses on testing sociological hypotheses with respect to inequalities and social stratification (Kapilashrami, & Meer, 2015), socialization, social values and norms (Mackenbach, 2016; Karnoven *et al.*, 2018), thus contributing to the analysis of health institutions and health policies. Such analysis is central in examining emergent themes, such as the health of vulnerable groups and international comparisons of social inequalities and quality of care. It is within this set of studies that the role of technology has gained special attention.

Early studies on technological determinism or the impact of technology on society (Postman, 1954) identified technology or technological advances as the central causal element in processes of social change (Croteau & Hoynes, 1967). As a particular technology becomes stable, its design tends to dictate users' behaviors, consequently diminishing human agency. There are two types of technology determinism: *hard determinism* and *soft determinism*. According to the *hard determinism* perspective, technology emerges regardless of social concerns and creates an institutional force of its own that shapes social norms and behaviors. Its autonomous activation serves the interests of technology-oriented agents, and individuals cannot control its outcomes. This perspective, however, overlooks the social and cultural circumstances in which the technology was developed. In contrast, *soft determinism* in technology is a moderate perspective, which posits that technology agents leave enough space for individuals to decide how technology is used and how its outcomes are defined.

One form of technological determinism is media determinism, a philosophical and sociological standpoint, according to which the media have the power to impact society. The theory of technological determinism in media gained attention when Marshall McLuhan's statement, *"the medium is the message"* became a central theme in technology studies for describing the essence of civilization. McLuhan (1962) later claimed that not all types of technology matter and that in the area of communication, only certain communication media can significantly affect social behaviors. Extending this line of thought, the media ecology perspective suggests that new forms of media communication technology may become the main framework that will facilitate the implementation of a wide range of social norms and behaviors (Chipidza & Leidner, 2019; Gencarelli, 2006), including health behaviors (Verhoeven & Tonkens, 2013). In fact, the more information and communication technologies (ICT) penetrate the lives of individuals, the more likely they will become more engaged in technology-based information, with the intensity and wide range of ICT crosscutting national and international borders (Verhoeven & Tonkens, 2013; Amnå, 2012). In nations that invest more in technology, the flow of information will be more intense and the odds of higher exposure to health issues will be greater (Chaeyoon & Sander, 2013; Jho & Song, 2015; Carty, 2010). This trend will affect existing institutions that organize support for and further develop new technology (Lenzi *et al.*, 2015).

Indeed, the expanded influence and expansion of ICT in society has led to the *normalization hypothesis*. This hypothesis posits that when *technology* affects the processes through which practices become routinely embedded in everyday life and implemented across a range of individuals' life. These processes will gradually become fully embedded, even in previously conflicted areas of social interactions that are of primary importance (May & Finch, 2009; Kim & Zhang,

2015). In fact, the Media-System Dependency theory, suggests that "the more a person depends on having his or her needs met by media use, the more important will be the role that media play in the person's life, and therefore the more influence those media will have on the person" (p. 273). As a result, the rise of the information society and the adoption of the Internet will reduce social inequalities because accessing and using the Internet at home and at work can increase access to services, including health services (Mesch *et al*., 2012).

The social stratification perspective maintains though, that the use of technology will benefit primarily those who already have better resources, therefore amplifying existing social inequalities (Chen *et al*., 2014; Neves *et al*., 2018). Internet use among advantaged groups will expand their social capital and consequently enhance their position of domination in society (Rosenberg, 2020). This is why knowing how to create and use technology needs to be connected with social processes at the time when socially bound knowledge is introduced and advanced and should find expression in how other institutions change and adapt to evolving situations (Mano, 2015; Mesch, 2016).

The interactive play between technology and social institutions facilitates making adjustments in use according to how individuals respond to technology innovations. Indeed, as opposed to hard and soft technology determinism approaches, the *social determinism* approach suggests that social circumstances "select" which technologies are adopted, while technology intertwines with implicated social processes. This interplay has led to the development of a novel approach to the use of online health information and access to online health forums. Known as social construction of technology (also referred to as SCOT), this approach contends that no technology can determine human action, but rather that human action shapes how technology is used. This is because technology is "embedded" in different social contexts, and different groups will use technology in various ways and to different extents (Rosenblum *et al*., 2017). As a result, the degree that technology is adopted necessitates that individuals are in favor of its use.

MEDIA THEORIES OF TECHNOLOGY ADOPTION

The Technology Acceptance Model (TAM) (Davis, 1989) is a general model that considers how variations in accepting computerized technology reflect a set of facilitating conditions, including expected effort, performance and social influence (Al-Ali & Haddad, 2004; Venkatesh & Bala, 2008). First, individuals will adopt technology when they assess its perceived usefulness and perceived ease of use as high. In fact, existing studies suggest that individuals who are skilled in and/or accustomed to using mobile devices, as is often the case with the younger generation, are more likely to identify with a perspective that justifies, enhances and expands the use of mobile technology. Second, ICT use shapes a new set of attitudes regarding technology's potential to contribute to health purposes. These attitudes not only reflect individuals' personal experiences prior to using mobile health applications, but their overall evaluations of technology as well. Such attitudes are likely to further enhance technology use (Ahadzadeh *et al.*, 2015; Chung & Koo, 2015).

Another perspective in technology adoption is the *Uses and Gratifications Theory* (UGT), which focuses on how differences in motivation affect the extent of technology use (Coyne *et al.*, 2015; Elhai *et al.*, 2017). Individuals seek to attain objects and processes to meet their needs and goals. Variations in motivation stem from many factors, among them age (Coyne *et al.*, 2015), personal inclinations (Mano, 2014) entertainment (Rokito *et al.*, 2019) and health (Mano, 2019). The main gratification categories are:

- *content gratification* stemming from accessing the right information;

- *process gratification* stemming from the satisfaction in using a particular media form;

- *social gratification* stemming from creating and vitalizing social relationships.

A higher level of gratification is likely to increase the *perceived functionality* of mobile health applications, while familiarity with mobile health applications will increase their level of use and the need to update them (Ranck, 2016). Underlying this approach are the assumptions of the *Social Diversification Hypothesis* (Mesch, 2007; Mesh *et al.*, 2012).

The Social Diversification Hypothesis (hereafter SDH) expands the theoretical background provided by the aforementioned communication and technology approaches, illustrating how application of a social science perspective increases our potential to compare the sociability patterns of individuals and communities (Mesch, 2007; Mesh *et al.*, 2012). Since ICT serves as a low-cost medium (Bundorf *et al.*, 2006; DiMaggio & Bonikowski, 2008), the use of health-related communication can expand the alternatives available to sociable individuals for entering into an extended span of social interactions, providing an additional source of health information despite geographic distance and time gaps. Clearly, then, ICT lowers the barriers to accessing health information and facilitates higher health literacy among disadvantaged groups, thus increasing their motivation to use ICT for an expanded range of services (Sillence *et al.*, 2007). SDH remains skeptical about these assumptions and is concerned with differential use of ICT according to people's social position in society, positing that ICT adoption may replicate or even amplify existing social inequalities. Inherent in SDH is the notion that individuals differ in their ability to gain access to social services, as services reflect residential and social capital (Korup & Szydlik, 2005; Mano, 2016). These skeptical assumptions are partially addressed by theories focusing on individual-level psychological aspects of technology adoption. Health adoption models test these assumptions.

BEHAVIORAL MODELS OF ONLINE HEALTH USES

The behavioral approach to online health uses necessitates the introduction of psychological components addressing the link between technology and health behaviors.

Health Belief Model

The *Health Belief Model (hereinafter: HBM)* applies the concepts of self-efficacy and health empowerment to examining health beliefs. It was originally developed for predicting the performance of screening behaviors and vaccinations (Redding *et al.*, 2000), but since then it has been used to explain other behaviors. The HBM incorporates two categories of relevant effects in health-related technology adoption:

(1) The category of *perceived threats to health* (Ahadzadeh *et al.*, 2015; Akompab *et al.*, 2013) addresses the importance of evaluating perceived risks of health threats (Redding *et al.*, 2000). This concept reflects the degree of perceived susceptibility (also referred to as vulnerability) and perceived severity of health concerns. Individuals exhibiting this vulnerability may need to assess the likelihood of contracting a disease or developing a particular behavior. This necessitates to evaluate the vulnerability of close family members facing a history of disease and the likelihood of a close partner contracting a disease (Ahadzadeh *et al.*, 2015; Jones *et al.*, 2014).

(2) The category of *behavior evaluation* includes the perceived benefits and perceived barriers of carrying out a particular health-improving behavior (Lajunen & Rasanen, 2004). The benefits refer to the perceived effectiveness of performing or changing a behavior, while the barriers refer to the perceived costs or obstacles in doing so (Redding *et al.*, 2000). *Perceived usefulness* refers to the belief that the adopted technology helps individuals perform a task better. *Perceived ease of use* is the belief that technology can be used with little or no effort, especially in m-Health, eHealth and telemedicine research (Or *et al.*, 2011; Keselman *et al.*, 2008).

Health Empowerment Model

Empowerment is a general term that captures the transition from a state of powerlessness to a state of relative control over any specific aspect of an individual's life. Health empowerment is often considered to be the "holy grail of health promotion" (Rissel, 1994). The Health Empowerment Perspective explains the empowering effect of information (Lemire *et al.*, 2008; Mano, 2014a), such that its consumers become pro-active in terms of health care (Rains, 2007). This empowerment finds expression in better and more equal relationships with health professionals (HPs) (Caiata-Zufferey *et al.*, 2010), better decisions regarding one's own health and adopting or changing one's health behavior (Mano, 2014a, 2014b; McKinley & Wright, 2014).

Online searches for health information satisfy two purposes: *functionality*, because online health searches cover a wide range of issues and enable selective processing, channel complementation and more (Dutta & Bodie, 2008; Mesch, 2011), and *gratification*, because online information-seeking improves the user's level of knowledge about health concerns (Dutta-Bergman, 2004b, 2006). According to Bandura's self-efficacy hypothesis (1997), health can be promoted by social cognitive means (Bandura, 2004). When people believe they can produce desired effects by their actions, they have higher incentive to act or persevere in the face of difficulties (Dutta-Bergman, 2004c). As individuals become more conscious of health concerns, they are more likely to search for health information for themselves as well as for family members and friends (McKinley & Wright, 2014), leading to a higher level of health empowerment. Indeed, having a defined purpose when seeking out information is important. Yet there is a difference between seeking a specific type of background information about a particular medication and searching through a list of possible sources for a more detailed description of a disease (Dutta-Bergman, 2004d). Reports indicate that 56% of online users look for information about new treatments and medications (Fox & Connolly, 2018; Rana & Dwivedi, 2015; Rana *et al.*, 2015).

In fact, health information-seekers, whether intentionally or not, are interested in increasing their level of empowerment toward some kind of health change. The Internet is a convenient medium that is easily accessed and provides a wide range of options for all individuals. Online health information seems to offer an efficient means of attaining health information (best process), although not necessarily in the most effective manner (best outcome). In this case, knowing that the Internet is a reliable source of information triggers a process that promotes attainment of the necessary resources and skills. When individuals reach a state of "critical consciousness" regarding the existing situation and when the resources are made available, the process is actualized and health outcomes can be attained (Shareef *et al*., 2011; Shaw & Sergueeva, 2019). In fact, the Internet is now regarded as a complementary source of health information rather than as a substitute for more traditional media sources (Mesch *et al*., 2012). Consequently, Dutta-Bergman (2006) differentiates between professional, consumer and community approaches (Dutta-Bergamn & Bodie, 2008).

The *professional approach* posits that empowerment is cultivated when individuals internalize aspects of health and disease, for internalization makes active engagement possible. This perspective implies that individuals search more for health-related information when they become more willing and are more likely to take an active role in preventing, attending to and following up on health issues (Salmond & Hall, 2003). The *consumer approach* suggests that information consumption leads to empowerment and increases the odds of making optimal decisions. Rational thinking is a basic prerequisite that enables individuals to exercise proper judgment in evaluating information and provides them the potential to process information through comparison with additional sources of information. The *community approach* suggests that community-based links, including virtual links, increase participants' potential to be exposed both to old and to new information as well as to the experiences of other members while providing opportunities to share personal experiences.

The relative weight of benefits *versus* barriers affects the likelihood of taking preventive action. When individuals perceive that the barriers are high, they are less likely to engage in healthy lifestyle behavior. The E(extended) HBM model (Bylund *et al*., 2011) adopted notions from the health empowerment perspective to include cues to action and self-efficacy. Cues to action are environmental triggers that can motivate an individual to adopt a health-improving behavior or change an existing one (Akompab *et al*., 2013; Redding *et al*., 2000). Triggers can be both external (such as illness, death of a relative due to disease or information about the behavior or disease from media sources) and internal (health status) (Redding *et al*., 2000). All three behavioral approaches to health assume that having a defined purpose when seeking out information is important and that communicating personal needs (Fox *et al*., 2005) necessitates taking responsibility and posing questions and expects individuals' willingness to play an active role in preventing, treating and following up on health issues for themselves and others (Dutta-Bergman, 2006; Lee *et al*., 2018).

THE HEALTH ATTAINMENT PROCESS

The combination of sociological behavioral and ecological models of health showcases the existence of variations in health behaviors pointing to the complex nature of the health attainment process (Rosenberg, 2018). This study focuses on three types of actions sharing personal experiences regarding chronic health conditions (Kendall Roundtree, 2017), discussing the work of health institutions—a variation of posting reviews of doctors (Thackeray *et al.*, 2013), and posting or commenting on health-related content—a variation of "liking" or commenting on content provided by others (Kendall Roundtree, 2017). Similarly, Mano shows how differences between health attitudes and health behaviors are related to variations in the use of online health sources (Mano, 2019a; 2019b). In line with the well-established decision-making model (Adjen, 1983), we distinguish between (Mano, 2019);

- health attitudes
- health behaviors
- health changes

Health Attitudes

Online health-related activity may increase people's sense that their trust has been misplaced (Tustin 2010; Gibbons 2008), hence boosting their motivation to look for alternative health services/products/providers (Sciamanna *et al.*, 2004; Mccomas *et al.*, 2015), especially in the case of older individuals (Makai *et al.*, 2015). These motivations increase one's evaluations of positive health attitudes (Mano, 2018). Positive health attitudes about the online process affect one's choice about being treated by a specific physician, as well as the type of questions one asks when visiting a physician, such as questions relating to treatment type. In addition, drug recommendations are also affected by the extent of individuals' knowledge and the information they possess (Katz *et al.*, 2004), even when this information is of little or no relevance (Wagner *et al.*, 2004; Bundorf *et al.*, 2006).

Additional factors associated with health attitudes stem from the desire to change health habits, such as weight loss and smoking (Rice, 2006; Fox *et al.*, 2011). Being unable to attain physical access to a physician because of geographic distance or mobility restrictions can also affect health attitudes (Purcell & Fox, 2010). Nonetheless, gaps often emerge when information is not accompanied by intentions to use it to extend the scope of the search.

The *Theory of Reasoned Action* must be mentioned in this context (Redding *et al.*, 2000; Sutton, 2001; Venkatesh & Davis, 2000). According to this theory, the strongest predictor of an end behavior is the intention to perform it (Sutton, 2001). Among other things, this intention is shaped by attitudes towards technology (Redding *et al.*, 2000). The *Technology Acceptance Model* was developed based on this theory (Davis, 1989; Venkatesh & Davis, 2000; Venkatesh & Bala, 2008). In brief, this model posits that the more positive an attitude and the more importance others attribute to performing a behavior, the higher the intention to perform this behavior. Frequency of use and previous experience improve search skills, enabling users to place more trust in social media (McKinley & Wright, 2014; Park *et al*., 2009). Trusting the source of health information is important because health information accessed on the Internet may be misleading or misinterpreted, leading individuals to request inappropriate interventions and medications (Goodyear-Smith & Buetow 2001; Purcell & Fox 2010). Lack of consideration of and attention to the individual-level factors mentioned above will increase the risk of generating and deepening differences in access and use of eHealth and mHealth services (Iverson *et al*., 2008; Mano, 2016). For this reason, health institutions must address notions of effectiveness and efficiency in order to increase successful implementation of programs for illness prevention, early diagnosis and regular attention to leading a healthy lifestyle (Aceijas, 2011; Mattke *et al*., 2012).

Health Behavior

Health behavior includes several important factors: It involves channeling certain individual behaviors toward a goal within a time and content context. This channeling process reflects expected outcomes and motivations. When an individual's involvement is high, the level of health empowerment increases and so does the need for a higher level of involvement in health decisions, thus enabling individuals to make health changes (Dutta-Berman, 2008). An important assumption in this process is that accessing and using online health information affect users' health habits. Several studies have addressed differential needs and roles of technology for health purposes (Rosenberg *et al*., 2017) among patients diagnosed with cancer (Ahadzadeh *et al*., 2015), heart conditions (Kerr *et al*., 2010), diabetes (Pereira *et al*., 2015) and other long-term conditions (Kennedy *et al*., 2007; Rogers *et al*., 2011). *Perceived ease* of use is an important factor in these cases in the context of needing to perform daily routines, with the aim of lowering sources of dysfunction or sense of disease (Mano, 2015). Moreover, individuals' judgments of their ability to organize and adopt proper health behaviors must be adapted to designated types of performance (Bandura, 1986). This is especially important when using technology such as computers and smartphones.

Indeed, self-efficacy can trigger behavioral intention (Irani *et al*., 2009; Alalwan *et al*., 2015; 2016). Recent studies (Lim & Noh, 2017) show that self-efficacy promotes healthy behavior and the adoption of fitness applications. Fox and Connolly (2018) showed that self-efficacy exerts a positive influence on intentions to adopt mHealth applications. Nevertheless, in a more recent study Mano (2019) raises doubts regarding the extent to which self-efficacy is sufficient in introducing health behaviors. In fact, according to recent studies (Asimakopoulos *et al.*, 2017) neither general self-efficacy nor computer self-efficacy has any effect on participants' attitudes toward mobile fitness-tracking health technology and may even restrain individuals from adopting mHealth programs (Bhatnagar *et al.*, 2017). This may be why health empowerment stresses the importance of two types of motivations: a) general health-related searches that allow individuals to search on their own time and at their own pace and shape their understanding of their medical condition; and b) access to specific and relevant information that can increase chances of recovery because it allows individuals to eliminate sources of concern and misunderstandings, thus helping them gain a better perspective on a condition, treatment, or medication (Bandura, 1997, 2004).

Health Changes

Considering the topic of health changes as a communication issue suggests that individuals will be differentially affected by the use of online health information. Access to relevant information increases understanding, making it easier for individuals to acquire a complete perspective on their medical condition, treatment, or medication and thereby increasing their chances of recovery (Bandura, 2004). Indeed, individuals with specific medical conditions search for health and medical information about their condition in order to understand the symptoms and the side effects of a medication and even to search for alternative treatments. Easy access to a wide range of online forums and services, among them feedback, goal-setting and self-monitoring, has proven successful in addressing eating disorders (Azar *et al.*, 2013) and alcohol use disorders (Fowler *et al.*,2016), in encouraging physical activity (Coughlin *et al.*, 2016) and self-monitoring behaviors during weight loss (Rusin *et al.*, 2013), in recording food intake during weight loss programs (Hutchesson *et al.*, 2015) and in providing support in psychotherapy (Prentice & Dobson, 2014). Similarly, individuals with heart conditions (Kerr *et al.*, 2010), diabetes (Miller & Bauman, 2014; Pereira *et al.*, 2015), cancer (Mobasheri *et al.*, 2014) and other long-term conditions (Kennedy *et al.*, 2007; Rogers *et al.*, 2011) are more likely to make health changes to alleviate bothersome symptoms.

Health tracking behaviors include those that increase one's ability to monitor health concerns and detect early signs of health disturbances (Mano, 2015). Individuals will adopt rational behavior that reflects the benefits associated with the probability of adopting such behavior (Champion & Skinner, 2008). These changes can be also viewed along a risk-related nexus ranging from low risk to high risk (Mano, 2018; 2019). The effect of this approach was twofold: First, it led health policymakers and practitioners to reconsider the usability of digital tools in self-management practices for assessing clinical utility, benefits and risks, especially in the context of prevention and management of disease among those diagnosed with chronic conditions (Prentice & Dobson, 2014; Mosa *et al.*, 2012; Anglada-Martínez *et al.*, 2016). Second, it promoted further interest in public health and motivated communication studies that sought to assess the effect of online health forums on lifestyle and health-related changes (Mohaptra *et al.*, 2015). This is the reason why recent studies in public health adopt the ecological perspective that focuses on an integrative approach to health studies.

ECOLOGICAL MODELS

Individuals, groups, organizations and health systems play an important role in supplying health services and are significant agents in many aspects of service provision that generate health practices and effective health habits and changes among the service recipients (Schultze, 2005). Ecological models following this health perspective assume not only that multiple levels of influence exist but also that these levels interact and reinforce one another. This perspective is at the core of public health models and referred to as the social ecology perspective.

The ecological perspective assumes that individuals addressing health issues seek to be linked to other social entities in order effectively solve difficulties and concerns. As a result, individual are willing to adopt the concepts and ideas of others and to alter their behavior accordingly (Ronfenbrenner, 1979). Accordingly, the social ecology perspective proposes to link multiple levels of social interaction in issues of health. According to Stokols (1992, 1996), the social, physical, and cultural aspects of an environment have a cumulative effect on health. Stokols further contends that the environment itself is multilayered, since institutions and neighborhoods are embedded in the larger social and economic structures, and that the environmental context may exert a differential influence on the health of individuals, depending on their unique beliefs and practices. The social ecology framework for health research and practice is used to explain the etiology of a number of health problems. Social ecological analyses can also be useful in examining health problems in the context of life span developmental, sociodemographic, and societal circumstances that influence susceptibility to disease. Therefore, creating sustainable improvements in health is most effective when all of these factors are targeted simultaneously. Nevertheless, Stokols (1996) also notes that influencing all environmental aspects and all individual characteristics may be impractical. He therefore recommends focusing interventions on different levels of influence as well as considering the risks associated with the adoption of health behaviors (Mano, 2019). Indeed, social conditions in an individual's environment may impede the application of desired health regimes. This is why the **social ecology** can serve as a basis for developing educational, therapeutic, and policy interventions to enhance personal and community well-being (Stokols, 2000).

The ecology perspective suggests that searching for health information refer to a selectivity effect. Individuals who a priori are highly interested in health and medical issues are more likely to search for information because they must deal with their own health conditions more frequently (Purcell & Fox 2010; Dutta-Bergman 2004a). These individuals consider the possible effects of this decision on their condition. Some decisions have an impact on well-being, whereas others may have far-reaching consequences with respect to a particular medical issue. We must therefore distinguish between the goals shaping health decisions and health changes that affect (a) wellbeing, (b) health care and (c) chronic illness. Lifestyle behaviors include practices that increase the likelihood of feeling better through day-to-day routines, including exercise and better nutrition (Mano, 2014; 2016; 2019; Rosenberg *et al.*, 2020).

CHAPTER 2

Online Health Information Search and Epatients

The concept of patient engagement in health care has been gaining increasing attention, not only in the scientific literature but also as a requirement in the everyday practices of health care organizations. The growing body of literature devoted to patient engagement is mainly inspired by sociological and public health perspectives that have generated various theories and models to explain how people become active agents in their health and care management (Carman *et al.*, 2013, Guendalina *et al.*, 2018). This approach seeks to ensure that patients' needs, values, and preferences are taken into consideration (Matthys *et al.*, 2009). The emergence of e-patients plays an important role in this interactive process.

e-patients or "expert patients" are those who seek information and knowledge to solve their health needs, reflecting empowerment as "an active, participatory process through which individuals, organizations, and communities gain greater control, efficacy, and social justice" (Mo & Coulson 2014). e-patients are health consumers who come to their health providers armed with the information they found on the web (Ferguson, 2008). In many cases, these e-patients come to their health providers armed with the information they found on the web and preconceived notions about their diagnosis. They wish to participate actively in therapeutic decisions while relying on misleading or misinterpreted health information (Purcell & Fox, 2010). This select group of consumers has developed a sense of responsibility and willingness to be more involved in their health care. Yet, at the same time, in taking responsibility for their treatment, they are also more willing to challenge the authority of health care providers (Okun & Caligan, 2018; Mano, 2015) when these are not related to the line of thought adopted by their professional health provider.

INDIVIDUAL LEVEL EFFECTS

Online searching for health information reflects two aspects relevant to health attitudes: (a) degree of functionality: online health searches cover a wide range of sources and facilitate selective processing, channel complementation (Dutta and Bodie, 2008); (b) level of gratification: online information-seeking improves knowledge about health concerns (Dutta-Bergman, 2004b, 2006). Understanding why and whether, intentionally or not, e-patients are likely to trust their sources of information is highly significant, especially in the case of vulnerable individuals.

A large proportion of e-patients use online forums and social network sites to extract information about health care concerns and/or use the information to increase their knowledge about conditions of members belonging to the relevant group (Fox & Jones, 2009; Potts & Wyatt, 2002). People's capacity to attain health, for example, their ability to change health behavior, derives from access, collection, processing, and dissemination of appropriate information. Health information seekers are interested in increasing their level of empowerment so they can "consult" with their physicians armed with online information (Dutta-Bergman 2006; Murero & Rice 2006). Variations in the use of online health services and forums may derive from different motivations reflecting the degree to which individuals feel connected to a larger group (Yamamoto, 2011) and/or their trust in virtual communities (Hsu *et al.*, 2011). Individuals who are highly interested in health and medical issues from the outset are more likely to search for information, participate in online health-related groups, and feel more empowered as a result of acquiring and understanding health information (Dutta-Bergman, 2004a, 2004d). Individual empowerment can be associated with modern individualism and the reflexive construction of the "I" (Gidden, 1991).

According to media system dependency theory (Baran and Davis, 2000), "the more a person depends on having his or her needs met by the use of media, use the more important will be the role that media play in that person's life, and therefore the more influence those media will have on the person" (p. 273). Yet, according to Rissel (1994), individual-level empowerment should not be disconnected from the individual's social, political, economic, and cultural context because an individual cannot be seen as a context-free creature. In fact, empowerment as a collective and active participatory process enables individuals to exert more control over their environment (Mo & Coulson 2014). Examples of this may be found among patients who choose to avoid vaccinations based on extensive and possibly unsolicited and erroneous information on the internet (Mesch & Sverian, 2017). To one degree or another, these variations reflect relationships with institutional health care providers.

e-patients usually are younger and tend to be women. Women are more likely to have searched for health topics than men, and younger people tend to be better educated and belong to higher income groups (Rice, 2006; Fox & Jones, 2009).

In terms of health needs, health information-seekers on the internet can be grouped into three groups: healthy individuals, patients with chronic illnesses, and patients with acute illnesses who have a more acute need to search for information than others. Moreover, levels of technology skills distinguish between early and late adopters of technology. Indeed, as the pace of technology innovations increases, so does the probability that late adopters will probably face new and more demanding barriers (Barzilai-Nahon, 2006). Empirical findings suggest that for diseases such as heart disease, diabetes, and cancer, "sick-prone" groups differ from "healthy" groups in that "sick-prone" groups more likely to search for health-related information on the internet (Dutta-Bergman, 2006). A more important factor is the impact of online health information on the patient-physician relationship due to the high likelihood that a conscious patient who accesses health and medical information will attempt to break the knowledge monopoly traditionally assigned to doctors (Friedman *et al.*, 2014; Rogers *et al.*, 1997). Frequency and previous experience improve search skills, allowing users to trust social media (McKinley & Wright, 2014; Park *et al.*, 2009).

Autonomy, competence, and relatedness are often reported to be major factors in well-being. More important to health is the likelihood that individuals with higher autonomy levels will become more competent in fully interacting with others and sharing opinions in decision-making processes. These skills provide individuals with greater potential to cope with what is expected of them during health delivery processes, as in completing forms, for example (Nutbeam, 2008; O'Neil *et al.*, 2014). More importantly, these individuals are more likely to be more satisfied with health providers (Sharma *et al.*, 2017) and less discontent with health services provision (Street *et al.*, 2009). It is then that the patient-doctor relationship is associated with increased patient satisfaction. The result is adherence to treatment and continuity of care.

INSTITUTIONAL LEVEL EFFECTS

e-patients challenge and contradict the traditional physician-patient relationship (Lytle, 2017). They question the physician's monopoly on professional knowledge and are skeptical about previously held beliefs regarding the physician's exclusive access to medical knowledge (TIM, 2010; Diaz *et al.*, 2002). This leads to questioning the power relations between patients and physicians and necessitates more cooperation between the sides (Dutta-Bergman, 2006; Dutta & Boddie, 2008).

Three types of relationships between patients and health institutions emerge at the institutional level (Szasz & Hollender, 1956):

1. *Active-passive* describes a relationship in which the physician has full control over the relationship and the decision-making, as in the case of children and adults regarding medical treatments and procedures.
2. *Guided cooperation* describes a relationship in which the physician provides advice and makes recommendations but does not enforce cooperation so as to obtain consent for treatment, as in the case of teenagers.
3. *Mutual participation* describes a relationship in which patients and providers fully cooperate to reach and implement decisions about the patient's wellbeing.

The first two relationship types are associated with the authority-based or patriarchal model of physician-health consumer relationships (McKinstry, 2002). In the third type, the patient is regarded as a consumer, and the final decision is in the hands of the recipient, not the provider. The central assumption of this model is that the direction of the relationship between physician and patient emerges from differences in access to knowledge and information. In other words, health and medical information are resources that enable the "information control" that prevails in the medical profession (Waitzkin & Stoeckle, 1986). As a result of greater accessibility to these resources, the locus of power in health care is shifting, with physicians being asked to share their power with patients.

For an involving process to take place, doctors need to be educated in alternative strategies for handling e-patients with medical problems. Such strategies include presenting the pros and cons of different treatments and medications. This process entails a considerable amount of listening, which should be seen as an independent part of the consultation. Once the patient is involved, shared decision-making can begin. The process includes answering the patient's questions, soliciting the patient's preferences, and giving the patient-relevant and individualized information, ultimately leading to involving individuals in healthcare decisions concerning their own care (*van der Heide et al., 2015*). As noted in recent studies, approaching decision-making as a process instead of an event is in line with patient perspectives on patient involvement (Bodegïrd *et al.*, 2020). This type of involvement requires that the doctor be educated in alternative strategies for handling medical problems.

Indeed, these processes of information control (Ferguson, 2008) challenge institutional health care providers to adopt an equal role in their relations with their patients, who may challenge their authority. Healthcare providers need specific training to ensure that patient involvement is not compromised, especially in medically complex situations that entail more than one reason for the visit and/or include medical uncertainty. Physicians without proper training and experience may find such relationships challenging. As noted, seeing decision-making as a process rather than an event is in line with patients' perspectives on patient involvement (Bodegïrd *et al.*, 2020). Not surprisingly, searching for online sources of information is motivated by disappointment with information received from the institutional health setting. For all these reasons, providing information and listening to individuals' health concerns facilitate greater involvement of both parties in health decisions.

ONLINE HEALTH SERVICES

The provision of health services is an ongoing process. Health service costs are typically part of an annual budget cycle handled in terms of recurrent expenditures and not necessarily evaluated periodically (Streiner & Geoffrey, 2008). Existing general theories of services have been used to leverage the current eHealth discussion on how the internet can be harnessed to deliver healthcare outcomes (see Kelson *et al.*, 2017; Stellefson *et al.*, 2011). This approach to service costs creates problems in testing effectiveness levels (Schiavo, 2007), especially when health services include technology-mediated services (Mattke *et al.*, 2012). Boards of health usually follow four principles in setting standards that speak explicitly to public health capacity and in meeting the needs of local communities: 1) *Need* (how to address the population's health needs effectively and efficiently); 2) *Impact* (how to reduce health inequities); 3) *Capacity* (how to understand the local capacity and resources, including human resources, required to achieve outcomes); and 4) *Partnership and Collaboration* (how to foster partnerships to promote community capacities, *i.e.*, the system includes partners such as other agencies and non-governmental organizations).

According to Ashill *et al.* (2006), technology can elicit positive attitudinal and behavioral responses. Quality of life was tested among patients in Norway to examine the effect of remote monitoring. The results showed that online health services had no significant impact on the quality of life, suggesting that remote follow-up should be further explored as an option (Remedios López-Liria *et al.*, 2019). In another analysis, Tang, Yang, and Shao (2019) suggested modifying the technology acceptance model in health to incorporate measures of trust. Such modification would reduce the perceived risk to users so as to increase their acceptance of the service. For example, research evidence suggests that two technological solutions commonly introduced in hospitals have not improved patient safety measures. In fact, the provision of outputs and outcomes in the health sector is based on complex integration between human- and technology-based elements and is driven by high levels of professional and ethical guidelines. In this process, frameworks are lacking to address performance in the healthcare industry (Cozica, 2014). Hence, effectiveness criteria in health services are hard to define, reflecting the increasing significance of e-Health and m-Health on the micro-level (Mano, 2014, 2016).

TRUST

Trust is a key factor in any relationship and is critical for establishing and maintaining long-term relationships between service provider and customer (Doney & Cannon, 1997). Searching for health information online makes individuals more willing to transfer power from the institutional healthcare provider to the patient or the recipient of health consulting services. The motivation to search for medical and health information may initially be related to the extent to which the individual is satisfied with and trusts the health provider (Dutta, 2006). Evidence indicates that Internet users are likely to retain close contact with their physicians (Mano *et al.*, 2009; 2014). The more positive the attitude of these users and the more satisfied are with the physician the more likely it is that e-patients will be willing to adopt a particular health behavior and the greater their intentions to carry out the behavior. Sharing medical decision challenges people's "blind" trust in medical authorities and leads to a shift toward "informed" trust that results in higher health empowerment (Dutta-Bergman, 2006; Murero & Rice 2006) since e-patients search the internet and consult their physician armed with information (Dutta- Bergman, 2006; Murero & Rice, 2006; Purcell & Fox, 2010; Lustria *et al.*, 2011).

Expressions of lack of trust dissatisfaction are important components of the health information control process (Ferguson, 2008). Yet even those who are aware of health information exert only minimal efforts in improving their health, regardless of whether they access health services online. Indeed, some minority groups can even express mistrust (Gibbons, 2008; Mesch *et al.*, 2012). Hence, trusting the source of health information is important because health information accessed on the Internet may be misleading or misinterpreted, leading individuals to request inappropriate interventions and medications (Goodyear-Smith & Buetow 2001; Purcell & Fox 2010). Hence, *dissatisfaction with institutional health care provider*s is often a factor that pushes individuals to consider preferring online health information (Mano, 2014) and SNS sources (Rosenberg *et al.*, 2019). This is especially true in that increasing skills, ongoing network health-related activity, more accessing and writing of blogs, and use of various health sites increase the level of online dependency. Individuals often seek information about a treatment, a specific physician or a particular institution for themselves or other family members and friends.

Self Determination Theory (SDT) is helpful in understanding variations in individuals' trust levels. Recent studies have shown that actors, barriers, facilitators, and demographic characteristics influence whether and how patients disclose online health information during consultations. These studies discuss the mechanisms through which online information can influence patients' relationships with their physicians (Mano, 2015). Patients who seek information on a health topic may find it difficult to gauge the reliability of a webpage. Indicators of quality aim at guiding patients toward high caliber information. Core indicators directly assess information quality. In fact, people who have trouble evaluating online health information may receive erroneous or incomplete information. Such information has been shown to be related to adverse health outcomes, such as low participation in screening programs or low adherence to treatments (Allegrante *et al.*, 2019).

Not surprisingly, trusting online health information has become a source of concern due to potential sources of disinformation in internet health information-seeking behavior. This concern reflects both the immediate impact on individuals' health and wellbeing as well as the long-term impact on their relationships with physicians. Studies show that patients indeed use the information they find online to prepare themselves for doctor visits and bring this information to the consultation. Appropriate responses to this information can help make it personally meaningful, potentially increasing patient involvement in decision-making (De los Reyes, 2019). The effect of online health-related activity on individuals' motivation leads individuals into looking for alternative health services, products, and providers, especially when the extent of dissatisfaction with the institutional health care provider is significant (Mano *et al.* 2009; 2015).

Hence, trust is a fundamental part of health delivery and is considered to be a precondition for cooperation (Gambetta, 1988). When people question the physician's monopoly on professional knowledge, they become skeptical about previously held beliefs regarding physicians' exclusive access to medical knowledge (TIM, 2010; Diaz *et al.*, 2002). This causes them to question the trust as well as the power relations between patients and physicians, thus necessitating more cooperation between the sides (Dutta-Bergman, 2006; Dutta & Boddie, 2008). In fact, blind trust may occasionally facilitate poor care but overrated trust involves risk-taking in cases when the actions of one party can affect the other in sharing information and ideas and addressing concerns. This is possibly the reason why trust challenges the traditional physician-patient relationship and increases the importance to understand the needs of health consumers (Dang *et al.*, 2017).

CHAPTER 3

Social Media and Social Networks For Health Purposes

In affluent post-industrial societies, online information has expanded rapidly over time, providing easy and inexpensive access to information and other people (Bundorf *et al.*, 2006; DiMaggio & Bonikowski, 2008; Graham & Dutton, 2018). Communication on health issues is growing as more and more people go online to interact with others having the same or similar health conditions (Greene *et al.*, 2010; Li, 2013). This new state of connectivity has expanded and even replaced traditional modes of communication. It has increased people's interest in health changes and in dietary and wellbeing routines and has made them aware of existing health alternatives that find expression on both the micro and macro levels of online health services and online forums. Considering the importance of these new forms of connectivity and influence on everyday life activities, institutional health providers have gradually adopted the use of virtual platforms to increase the involvement of individuals in their health care management.

The rapid increase in the number of users of online health information has been accompanied by the development of health-related expectations and attitudes towards health and has facilitated the emergence and expansion of groups interested in health (Chen & Lee, 2014) both among individuals with health concerns and among those without such concerns. The literature mentions three main types of health participation activities: sharing personal experiences regarding chronic health conditions (Kendall Roundtree, 2017); discussing the work of health institutions, usually by means of posting of reviews about doctors (Thackeray *et al.*, 2013); and posting or commenting on health-related content (Palsdottir, 2014) and even on "expert" information.

Health-related information exchange (Thoren *et al.*, 2013) has led to the establishment of health communities such as Patients Like Me (Murthy *et al.*, 2011) and health-related groups on Facebook (Greene *et al.*, 2010) and Twitter (Murthy *et al.*, 2011; Zhang *et al.*, 2013).

Social media (SM) refer to the collective use of online communication channels dedicated to community-based input, interaction, content-sharing and collaboration. Social media reflect the symbiotic relationship between producing and consuming online content as well as the combined outcomes of globalization and networking.

The importance of social media emerges from the mass transition to the information era in the wake of the shift from traditional economies and the industrial revolution to the generation of global economies based on the amount of information available *via* technologies such as computers. The power inherent in social media reflects the potential of mass communication for exchanging worldviews, products, ideas and other cultural elements on virtual devices. In the United States, about seven out of ten individuals use social media to connect with others, receive news content, share information, and entertain themselves (Pew Research Center, 2018). Yet, the effectiveness of social media for healthcare remains inconclusive, with contradictory evidence from different countries (Twenge *et al.*, 2018).

The impact of social media has been synchronous with the introduction of Web 2.0 platforms, which have generated a social phenomenon known as prosumption. Prosumption reflects the symbiotic relationship between producing and consuming online content. Individuals with network access and skills can obtain a vast amount of informative content without leaving their homes. With a single click they have immediate access to many sources of information whose content is available and constantly updated in different languages and formats. This content can offer different perspectives and opinions on the same topic (Miller & Bell 2012; Riggare *et al.* 2017).

Social media can offer individuals a platform that overcomes barriers of distance and time, enabling them to connect and reconnect with others and thereby expand and strengthen their offline networks and interactions (Antoci *et al.*, 2015; Hall *et al.*, 2018; Subrahmanyam *et al.*, 2008). The use of SM has indeed successfully reached the health domain, mostly because SM helps people achieve a better perspective about health problems (Mano, 2014a). The ability to connect with others who have similar health conditions (Greene *et al.*, 2010; Li, 2013) has increased the impact of health-related online forums and social networks in providing social support and "expert" information. This interaction has generated active and collaborative creation (Scanfeld *et al.*, 2010) and updating of health content (Kaplan & Haenlein, 2010). SM applications include blogs, social networking sites such as Facebook, content-sharing sites such as YouTube and more (Househ *et al.*, 2014). As a result, health communities such as Patients Like Me (Murthy *et al.*, 2011) and health-related groups on Facebook (Greene *et al.*,

2010) and Twitter (Murthy *et al.*, 2011) have been established. Clearly the use of social media is especially meaningful for individuals facing health concerns.

The rapid integration of social media into everyday communication, including social network sites and weblogs, offers new sources of information that have become evident in the workplace (Skeels & Grudin, 2009), in entertainment and culture (Kim *et al.*, 2010; Zheng, 2014), in social change (Kim *et al.*, 2010) and in health (Korda & Itani, 2013; Li, 2013; Newman *et al.*, 2011; Zhang, 2013; Bekalu *et al.*, 2019). Social media have helped create social networks which have facilitated the formation and development of social capital. Through the social networks available online, people can share their ideas, knowledge and apprehensions with people who have experienced the same problem. Online discussion networks that discuss cases or symptoms experienced by patients with similar problems have the potential to bring about improvements in health and to promote greater patient autonomy. This capacity enables users to develop and disseminate their own content (Benetoli *et al.*, 2018) and to communicate (Alas *et al.*, 2013) effectively regardless of place and time (Antheunis *et al.*, 2013, p.426).

Individuals who have access to the network and the skills to handle this tool can obtain a vast amount of informative content. Without leaving home, they can access many sources of information at any time with a single click. The content they access is updated continuously, available in different languages and formats, and can provide different perspectives and opinions on the same topic (Miller & Bell 2012; Riggare *et al.* 2017). Through WIFI routes, the internet has become available in all places and at no cost, enabling users to develop and disseminate their own content (Benetoli, Chen & Aslani, 2018) and to communicate (Alas *et al.* 2013) efficiently in terms of place and time (Antheunis *et al.*, 2013, p.426). In line with this contention, Moretti and Barsottini (2017) observed that participation in social networks has the potential to improve patients' social life and reduce their sense of hopelessness. Indeed, the internet has transformed researching health information from an uncommon practice to one that is part of the daily routine of many individuals (Holmes *et al.* 2017).

This social capital, in turn, allows individuals to capitalize on the resources of other network members, for example in the form of information and social support (Viswanath, 2008). Social networks are therefore linked to a variety of positive social outcomes such as trust and reciprocity that engender better health (Ellison *et al.*, 2007; Nabi *et al.*, 2013; Nieminen *et al.*, 2013). Social networks serve to support people and relationships that are separated by time, geographic location and/or even cultural and group identification characteristics. By increasing the proximity between members in the virtual space, social networks enable connected individuals to create a strong support system based on a weak connection. By doing so, they increase the potential of participants to express unusual and possibly conflicting views (Burt, 2009). Hence, social networking transforms originally weak ties into stronger ties and is a convenient way of reinforcing older connections as well.

Indeed, the internet has transformed researching health information from an uncommon practice to one that is part of the daily routine of many individuals (Holmes *et al.* 2017).

People go online to interact with others having the same or similar health conditions (Greene *et al.*, 2010; Li, 2013). Using online discussion networks to identify with cases or symptoms experienced by patients with similar problems can provide improvements in health and promote greater patient autonomy. Following this line of thinking, Moretti and Barsottini (2017) claim that participation in social networks can improve a patient's social life and reduce hopelessness. Thus, health-related online forums and social networks provide people opportunities for social support and information exchange. Indeed, health communities such as Patients Like Me (Murthy *et al.*, 2011) and health-related groups on Facebook (Greene *et al.*, 2010) and Twitter (Murthy *et al.*, 2011) (Thoren, *et al.*, 2013) are highly instrumental in providing emotional support, information and advice (Zhang *et al.*, 2013; 2017).

According to Ferguson (2008), access to internet information changes individuals from "passive" recipients of health services to "active" seekers of health information. More importantly, they gain access to and begin to use these forums and social media (Greene *et al.*, 2010; Murthy *et al.*, 2011) and forums (Savolainen, 2011; Greene *et al.*, 2010; Li, 2013). Understanding the effectiveness of social media for health purposes necessitates first understanding the extent to which the individuals who use SM are satisfied with technology (Allegrante & Auld, 2019). Deng *et al.* (2019) suggested that when users are satisfied, they tend to continue using the services (Ghobakhloo *et al*, 2019). The impact of satisfaction is also evident among patients using health portals, where satisfaction indicates the need to use. Health portals motivate patients to use technology because they offer a principal source of direct contact with health providers who are important to that individual (Christakis & Fowler, 2013). Social media use in contrast to the digital divide hypothesis is not associated with education, race/ethnicity or income. Hence, a large segment of the adult population can effectively use and be reached though social media (Harris *et al.*, 2013). Indeed, health-related online communication has increased exponentially among individuals with or without health concerns.

The major types of these activities include sharing personal experiences (Kendall Roundtree, 2017), reporting on the quality of health institutions and health personnel (Thackeray *et al.*, 2013), and focusing on health-related products and services (Palsdottir, 2014). The rapid expansion of the number of online health information users has been accompanied by the rapid development of health-related expectations and attitudes towards health and has facilitated the emergence and expansion of groups interested in health (Chen & Lee, 2014).

The reinforcement provided by social media has encouraged increased access to information and the adoption of health behaviors aimed at attaining and maintaining healthy lifestyles (Centola, 2010; Mano, 2018; 2019). Indeed, social media can offer additional perspectives on health problems (Mano, 2014a). These experiences have become part of the daily activities of many individuals (Holmes *et al.*, 2017). However, the probability that individuals will behave in a specific way is not a direct outcome of social media use because according to the lifestyle/exposure theoretical framework (Lam & Mesch, 2017; Mesch, 2009), health behaviors need to address lifestyle and personal habits (Mesch, 2000; Lam & Mesch, 2017; Mesch, 2009; Dodel & Mesch, 2018). For this reason, we now examine existing differences in behaviors in relation to variations in socioeconomic background (Lam & Mesch, 2017).

SOCIOECONOMIC VARIATIONS IN USE OF SOCIAL MEDIA

Age Effects

Age is a central factor in social media studies. For example, the association between technology and adolescent well-being has yielded controversial findings, with some studies highlighting the potential dangers of this association (*e.g.*, Twenge *et al.*, 2018; Wartella & Robb, 2008) and fewer studies calling attention to its promises (*e.g.*, George & Odgers, 2015; Gray *et al.*, 2005; Mills, 2016). Indeed, evidence suggests that technology use may serve to meet certain developmental needs (Borca *et al.*, 2015). For instance, adolescents employ technology in an effort to develop close and meaningful relationships (Reich *et al.*, 2012; Valkenburg & Peter, 2011), explore their identity (Subrahmanyam *et al.*, 2006), and find information about developmentally sensitive issues (Valkenburg & Peter, 2011). Research shows that more than 80 percent of young adults use social media (Perrin, 2015; Smith & Anderson, 2018) for at least an hour every day (Nielsen, 2018).

Some estimates suggest that the use of social media among 44% of U.S. adults between the ages of 19 and 32 is related to addictive characteristics that prevent participation in normal life activities (Shensa *et al.*, 2017). Moreover, some research has found that social media use can lead to stress (Beyens *et al.*,2016), difficulties with emotion regulation (Hormes *et al.*, 2014; Twenge *et al.*, 2019) and even problems with self-image (Tiggemann & Slater, 2013) and physical and psychological health (Rosen *et al.*, 2014; Twenge *et al.*, 2018; Duvenage *et al.*, 2020). The ubiquitous and continuous state of being connected to digital media has been referred to in terms of "constancy" issues Borzekowski (2019), reflecting variations in aging processes.

The term aging is used to describe the process of getting older. Successful aging takes into consideration the physiological, psychological and sociological concerns of older citizens. Today's higher life expectancy shapes physical and psychological expectations for a better quality of life and wellbeing. Social media have had a positive influence on older individuals. Interaction on social media enables them to be active in creating (Scanfeld *et al.*, 2010) and updating health content collaboratively *via* blogs, social networking (Facebook), and content-sharing (YouTube) (Househ, Borycki & Kushniruk, 2014). Recent studies (*e.g.*, Bordes *et al.*, 2020) have shown how social media platforms provide viable options or complement traditional face-to-face contacts with healthcare providers, thus serving as a necessary patient support system. Through their into social routines often observed in various health interventions (Duvenge *et al.*, 2020), social media have helped improve dietary habits (Power *et al.*, 2019) and increased the effectiveness of promoting postpartum weight loss among low-income groups (Reading *et al.*, 2019). Nonetheless, older users consistently report that the needs of older cohorts are different (Subrahmanyam *et al.*, 2008; Gibson *et al.*, 2010; Chou *et al.*, 2012; Norval, 2012; Rasmussen *et al.*, 2020).

Gender Effects

The issue of gender in health-related use of the internet has been well documented in studies in the fields of internet sociology and public health (Lee *et al.*,2014; Mano, 2016). The most stable finding across studies is that female users search for health information more than male users (Chen & Lee, 2014; Lee *et al.*, 2014; Mesch *et al.*, 2012), while male users are more active health participants than female users (Mano, 2019). The explanation for these consistent findings can be found in the traditional role of women in issues related to health, both within and outside the family (Lee *et al.*, 2014). Yet women are not necessarily more likely to use online health services and online forums of health (Mano, 2016).

Understanding the influence of technology-embedded communication in terms of "friendly" or "unfriendly" means of communication (Wacjman, 2004; Van Dijk & Peters, 2010) is an important theoretical perspective in developing hypotheses about the way gender may sustain or block exposure and use (Shashaani, 1997; McAndrew & Jeong, 2012). Such differences may affect women's willingness to use mobile health applications to access health services, since knowledge about health risks and benefits for different health issues is a strong predictor of an individual's need to exercise control over health practices, especially when health concerns are present. Thus, gender can moderate the "perceived functionality" of mobile health applications.

Gender is also related to the way information is evaluated in terms of its practicality, cost and effectiveness in daily activities (Mano, 2014, 2016). This has been explained by women's unique cognitive functioning and communication style (Eagly, 2005; Kelan, 2008). Women are more likely to be selective in processing information (Dutta & Bodie, 2008; Mesch *et al.*, 2012) seeking to reach a higher level of "gratification" regarding health concerns (Dutta-Bergman, 2004b, 2006). This is even more amplified for women diagnosed with cancer because they must cope with various health-related functions on a daily basis to address their health-related concerns. Moreover, women have been shown to be highly discerning about the scope of their internet use. They are likely to search different sites than men (Kim *et al.*, 2007) and to use information in different ways (Large *et al.*, 2002; Lewis, 2006) and for several persons, including family and community members (Katz *et al.*, 2004; Rice, 2006; Bianco *et al.*, 2013).

Health Status

The use of technology devices is considered a significant means of self-management because it facilitates treatment and follow-ups and prevents unnecessary health complications (Bianco *et al.* 2013; Renahy *et al.* 2008). According to the Health Belief Model (HBM), the impact of perceived threat (Ahadzadeh *et al.*, 2015) and the benefits associated with the probability of adoption of such behavior are evaluated by a set of constructs (Champion & Skinner, 2008). For the most part, the association between HBM constructs and outcomes has been validated with gender-mixed samples (Gerend & Shepherd, 2012; Mano, 2016). The consensus is that the higher the perceived threat, the greater the benefits. Moreover, the lower the impact of barriers, the higher the probability of engaging in preventive behavior or in changing behavior to address health concerns, especially when the benefits outweigh the barriers (Mano, 2019).

Nevertheless, recent evidence indicates that chronic disease (CD) does not necessarily increase the use of technology devices to seek health services (Jiang *et al.* 2007; Mano 2014; Mesch *et al.* 2012). On the one hand, having a CD increases the odds of seeking health information online (Dutta-Bergman 2006; Mano 2014a). Moreover, the use of technology devices increases the odds of monitoring a health problem in time if medical appointments have been delayed and provides timely access to lab test results (Purcell & Fox 2010; Lustria *et al.*

2011; Mano 2014b; Bundorf *et al.*, 2006; Mano 2014b; Manhattan Research 2013). The benefits of communicating with healthcare providers and/or website moderators to receive feedback and social support and tracking (*e.g.*, graphical displays of uploaded personal data) were shown to be particularly useful for self-management support but less so for improvements in medication adherence, biological outcomes and healthcare utilization (Ezendam *et al.*, 2013).

On the other hand though, searching for health information does not necessarily encourage individuals to use online health services for self-care health management (Dutta and Bodie, 2008; Goldman & Smith 2011; Mano, 2014b). Some studies indicate that the use of technology devices to provide health services may lag behind the intended purposes and fail to provide effective health services (Chahal & Kumari 2012; Samoocha *et al.*, 2010; Betancourt, 2015; Manhattan Research, 2013). Existing studies indicate that individuals with CDs do not necessarily access virtual services, especially patients diagnosed with cancer (Huang & Penson, 2008; Shim *et al.* 2006), heart conditions (Kerr *et al.* 2010), diabetes (Pereira *et al.* 2015) and other long-term conditions (Kennedy *et al.*, 2007; Rogers *et al.*, 2011).

Such empirical findings raise concerns regarding the extent to which the specific needs of CD patients are ignored or misunderstood (Betancourt, 2015), thus lowering the benefits of preventive online and offline health medical support (Betancourt, 2015; Seeman 2008; Manhattan Research 2013; Stellefson *et al.* 2013). In fact, these studies suggest that it may be likely that effective self-management of health does not eliminate the risk of hospital admission and of even higher mortality rates (Peterson *et al.* 2011). These risks may be related to differences in technology use. Evaluations are needed to determine the long-term effectiveness of social media services for more diverse samples of CD patients in order to translate new knowledge, social technologies and engagement techniques into "effective novel approaches for empowering, engaging, and educating older adults with chronic disease" (p. 265).

CHAPTER 4

Mobile Health Applications

The technological advancements in ICT have been mainly apparent in the use of smartphones and mobile internet. Indeed, this form of use has become prevalent in the everyday lives of smartphone and tablet users and has enabled consumers to access and share information on the go. Smartphone owners can choose from a wide-ranging assortment of messaging apps such as WhatsApp and can use mobile social media applications for travel, banking and avoiding traffic. Mobile health applications have been facilitated by the use of smartphones and other mobile communication devices. More than 3.4 billion smartphone and tablet users use mobile health applications. The use of these apps has enhanced individuals' health management, primarily because they are affordable and easy to use (Balapour *et al.*, 2019).

Mobile healthcare applications enable individuals to improve their state of healthcare (Veríssimo, 2018). Users of mobile health applications download and update health fitness programs, contact healthcare professionals and monitor health conditions. These apps improve medical data collection, medical service delivery, patient-doctor communication, and real-time monitoring and adherence support (Islam *et al.*, 2020). Most users access at least one health-related application (Krebs & Duncan, 2015). Evidence also supports the importance of social media and smartphones in facilitating communication exchanges with others who have similar health concerns (Scanfeld *et al.*, 2010; Church & de Oliveira, 2013), providing appointment reminders (Hocking *et al.*,2012) and encouraging the use of online health services (Mano, 2016a; Wu, *et al.*, 2007; Wu *et al.*, 2011).

In a recent study, 44% of the participants in a weight loss program chose to use their smartphones to record food intake. These participants reported greater adherence to self-monitoring behaviors during weight loss (Burke *et al.*, 2011; Rusin *et al.*, 2013; Recio-Rodríguez *et al.*, 2014; Dai *et al.*, 2020). Today the global mobile population totals 4 billion users and global mobile data traffic is expected to rise exponentially through at least 2022. Hence, it is not surprising that mobile communication technology has been called the "fastest diffusing medium on the planet ever" (Campbell, 2013:9).

Mobile health applications provide general support in the areas of preventative healthcare (de Jongh *et al.*, 2012), health monitoring (Luxton *et al.*, 2011; Mano, 2015, 2016) and illness management (Vodopivec-Jamsek, 2012; Mano 2016; 2018). Evidence shows that mobile health applications have been helpful for different health concerns. They provide feedback, goal-setting and self-monitoring in eating disorders (Azar *et al.*, 2013), alcohol use disorders (Fowler *et al.*, 2016) and in programs for stopping smoking (Ubhi *et al.*, 2016), encouraging physical activity (Coughlin *et al.*, 2015) and addressing issues during psychotherapy sessions (Prentice & Dobson, 2014).

Recent studies (Alalwan *et al.*, 2017) found that hedonic motivation, performance expectancy, effort expectancy, price value and trust are the main predictors of users' intentions to adopt mobile apps. Some mobile health applications such as Fitbit are especially designed to track patient health, while others can be used for fitness, cardiology, diabetes, obesity, stopping smoking, and chronic disease tracking for all age ranges (Lim & Noh, 2017; Silva *et al.*, 2015). Extrinsic/intrinsic motivation and technology constructs such as ease of use and usefulness have been expanded into novel constructs such as privacy concerns, risk beliefs, self-efficacy, autonomy and control (Fox & Connolly, 2018; Liu *et al.*, 2019; Zhao *et al.*, 2018).

Mobile health applications have been found effective in medical interventions (Rumsey & Harcourt, 2012) and attracted the attention of institutional healthcare providers (Ahad & Lim, 2014; Church *et al.*, 2013). Healthcare providers use mobile health applications for various purposes, including direct monitoring of patients, drug-referencing, decision support, electronic health records, medical education and more (Boulos *et al.*, 2014) reducing the number of times patients must visit the doctor because they enable at-home checkups (Mendiola *et al.*, 2015). These applications decrease the problems associated with shortage of time (Deng *et al.*, 2018). Some applications, such as InpharmD, enable professionals to make ad-hoc decisions and address issues regarding medication effectiveness, dosage and costs promptly (Wicklung, 2018). In that way, institutional health providers are able to decrease the pressure on professionals especially when individuals face chronic diseases (Quinn *et al.*, 2008).

Among the most notable of these applications are digital platforms for women providing ample support for fertility management, prenatal management and postpartum management. They also provide solutions facilitating the health of mother and child during the first six months. Other solutions include female diseases, such as breast cancer and menopause management. Due to their potential to enable self-monitoring these applications decrease the need to engage in time-consuming visits to professional clinics (Mendiola *et al.*, 2015). The use of applications has been particularly effective when complex health conditions are related to psychological difficulties (Rumsey & Harcourt, 2012; Normana *et al.*, 2019).

Yet, applications are seldom used as an alternative to traditional face-to-face contacts with healthcare professionals (Bessell & Moss, 2007). First, mobile devices present challenges for users in dealing with applications that require large amounts of computational resources (Dai *et al.*, 2020). Second, users' socio economic profile affects the quality of connectivity and higher expenses for updating smartphones and/or to fees for this high connectivity. For example, access to social media through smartphones and other connected technology has been found to be significantly lower among older adults, those with less education, and those with serious mental illnesses (Klee *et al.*, 2016). Third, the lack of tailored programs may lead to risks among individuals who lack health literacy or are relatively reckless (Mano, 2019).

Indeed, while it is reasonable to assume that institutional-level efforts should encourage the use of virtual health sources to increase health empowerment and self-management practices, considerable effort is now being invested in addressing individual-level constraints that play a significant role in the adoption of technology for health purposes. Individual-level constraints, among them lack of technology skills, chronic conditions and the gap between lifestyle and healthcare goals, prevent the effective use of eHealth and mHealth sources. As a result, and despite the potential benefits of mHealth apps, a number of reviews have highlighted their deficiencies, indicating that although these apps are often helpful, in some cases they may be detrimental to those who use them. Not many apps have been validated empirically (Bakker *et al.*, 2016), and those that have been evaluated are often unavailable to the public (Firth *et al.*, 2017; Parker *et al.*, 2018). Another concern about mHealth apps is their tendency to suggest that mental illness can be managed without treatment (Parker *et al.*, 2018). These concerns regarding the use of mobile health apps are both theoretical and methodological.

On the theoretical level, studies supporting the adoption of mHealth apps are based on considering mHealth in terms of the Theory of Reasoned Action (Fishbein & Ajzen, 1975; Zhang *et al.*, 2014), the Technology Acceptance Model (Davis, 1989; Deng *et al.*, 2018; Dou *et al.*, 2017) and the Unified Theory of Acceptance and Use of Technology (Hoque & Sorwar, 2017; Venkatesh *et al.*, 2003). The relatively restricted spectrum of these theories precludes the introduction of modifications. The social diversification hypothesis (Mesch *et al.*, 2014) and the technology identity theory (Carter & Grover, 2015) are of special relevance in analyzing new forms of technology (Kwon *et al.*, 2017; Lee & Cho,

2017; Lee *et al.*, 2017; Quaosar *et al.*, 2018; Yuan *et al.*, 2015). Inherent in both theories is the notion of push/pull decision-making (Mano, 2014) and the gap between lifestyle and healthcare practices (Mano, 2018; 2019; 2020; Antheunis *et al.*, 2013). These perspectives address a variety of individual health practices, ranging from simple lifestyle changes (Faiola *et al.*, 2018; Mano, 2016) to the self-management of chronic illnesses (Kaphle *et al.*, 2015; Petrovčič *et al.*, 2018).

On the methodological level, most existing studies are problematic for several reasons: (a) Many focus on specific groups, thus overlooking the fact that users are likely to face health-related situations that either encourage or deter further use of mobile health applications (Vaona & Schiavo, 2007; Mattke *et al.*, 2010; Braun *et al.*, 2017; Lupton, 2012). (b) The samples used in these studies are not representative of the target population in that they often comprise students or occasional app users who may or may not be patients (Kwon *et al.*, 2017; Lee & Cho, 2017; Lee *et al.*, 2017; Quaosar *et al.*, 2018; Yuan *et al.*, 2015). (c) Studies examining the use of mHealth do not consider the gaps between health skills and attitudes regarding the functionality of mobile health applications and disregard the immediate and remote outcomes and outputs of use (Mano, 2019). (d) The intensity and diversity of mobile health application use are also often overlooked. Heavy users consider the outcomes of mobile health application use to be more effective than do light and uncommitted users (Mano, 2018; 2019).

EVALUATIONS OF MOBILE HEALTH APPLICATIONS

Access to virtual health sources is associated with improved knowledge about health issues. Research has only recently begun to consider the strong impact of those sources on individuals and to assess the credibility and effectiveness of mHealth for health purposes. The market of applications devoted to well-being or lifestyle has grown to over 100,000, alerting mHealth institutional agents of safety to the lack of concrete definitions and sets of regulations governing the use of such apps (European Commission, 2016a). Healthcare institutions and professionals have begun to identify uncertainties and ambiguities in the use of commercial applications (Bijker 2010, p. 68). These authorities are expected to implement safety regulations and precedents to govern unsolicited use among individuals and patients without causing unnecessary damage to commercial development and progress in introducing new mobile health applications. General concerns also emerge because despite high accessibility and proven generalized beneficial effects on health routines, much remains to be learned from individuals' personal-level constraints. Indeed, increased use of mobile health applications by institutional healthcare providers (Chen *et al.*, 2017) has made it clear that the need to adopt such applications will grow over the next decades, leading to sustainable health improvements. Therefore, the adoption of mobile health technology is most effective when all these factors are targeted simultaneously.

Monitoring *Versus* Evaluation

Using mobile health applications without providing evidence of both monitoring and evaluation falls short of being considered adequate in terms of outcomes and outputs. In assessing mobile health applications, the literature distinguishes between two basic concepts: monitoring and evaluation.

a. Monitoring is a planned process of observation that closely follows a course of activities and compares what is happening with what is expected to happen. Periodic collection and review of information on program implementation, coverage and use and comparisons of this information with implementation plans help in identifying shortcomings before it is too late and provide criteria when progress is not properly attained.
b. Evaluation is a systematic process that assesses an achievement against preset criteria to determine the extent that the provided service needs and results are achieved and locate the reasons for any discrepancy. Evaluations seek to measure service relevance, efficiency and effectiveness. They measure whether and to what extent a program's inputs and services are improving the quality of people's lives.

Evaluation and monitoring are especially important for applications addressing the needs of individuals dealing with chronic conditions because they must assess the extent to which the use of a specific application was effective and delivered outputs in accordance with its objectives—as defined by the physician together with the individual (Bakker *et al.*, 2016). In the short term, individuals with a chronic condition will then be able to report that they are doing things differently. In the long term, however, these same objectives need to be evaluated by the institutional healthcare provider (Firth *et al.*, 2017a; 2017b; Parker *et al.*, 2018). If discrepancies emerge between individual and professional evaluations of mobile applications, further evaluations are necessary (Donker *et al.*, 2013; Parker *et al.*, 2018). Part of the problem derives from the fact that mobile health applications are not defined as medical instruments (Mantovani & Bocos, 2017). These discrepancies may lead to lowered trust in an app and even to its abandonment.

Knowledge that some apps may be harmful has spread rapidly, drawing attention to the special needs of individuals with health concerns (Mano, 2019). This has prompted greater integration between health, community and social service agents who promote the need for individuals to become more involved and responsible for their own care while overlooking issues related to individuals with low technical skills or to disadvantaged social groups (Mills *et al.*, 2017, Rosemberg *et al.*, 2019). This evidence points to the need to use a push/pull framework to evaluate applications, according to which individuals may either increase or decrease their reliance upon online sources of health information delivered virtually through eHealth and mHealth (Seth *et al.*, 2012; Mano, 2014).

mHealth applications have recently been clustered into nine clusters: General Health Informative, Institutional, Fitness, Physician Information, Mother and Child, Disease-Specific Care, Food and Nutrition and Homeopathic (Islam *et al.*, 2020). This clustering may increase the potential for adopting or deciding not to adopt a specific cluster of applications depending on people's individual and health needs. Research about the safety of these applications has led indeed to evidence indicating that reporting of safety concerns is needed to improve outcomes (Akbar *et al.*, 2020). Indeed, while participants in studies were generally enthusiastic, shared disease-related information and personal experiences and served as a source of education and peer support, they are often reported as lacking in traditional models of care (Des Bordes, *et al.*, 2020). This may explain why the concerns about the adoption of mHealth apps persist (Kwon *et al.*, 2017) and even increase when ethical aspects of the use rise.

In fact the rise of bioethics has expanded over the past few decades and includes now a variety of professional such as ethics consultants and leaders in public health institutions. policy. The role of these professional is to bring to light increased reflective thinking on the centrality of bioethicists so that the use of mobile technologies in health will accommodate for the increased needs of individuals without harming their safety and wellbeing. The assessment of mobile health applications will enable institutional healthcare providers to increase the quality of delivered health services and health programs, improve the likelihood of effective self-management practices and reduce the risk of inducing secondary digital divide effects. Indeed, ecological models assume the existence of multiple levels of influence that interact and reinforce one another (Nijman *et al.*, 2014; Terasse *et al.*, 2019).

In the future, apps should include follow-ups for improving treatment, diagnosing early symptoms, providing faster responses, accessing medical data and decision support systems, increasing digital health literacy and accentuating support on social platforms (Research 2 Guidance, 2017). It is that way that assessments of applications will increase the effectiveness levels of feasibility, functionality and clinical utility (Lupton, 2013; Mosa *et al.*, 2012; Prentice & Dobson, 2014; Husereau *et al.*, 2013).

COMMERCIAL HEALTH APPLICATIONS

Applications are used in a variety of contexts, and in the commercial spheres of activity applications are defined as self-contained, specialized programs generally accessed *via* a mobile device (*e.g.*, tablet or smartphone). A large proportion of these mobile technologies have created fundamental changes in practitioner workflow: dissemination of education from clinicians to patients, relay of self-assessment data from patients to providers, patient-provider interaction between visits, and patient engagement in care (Bakker *et al.*, 2016; Klasnja & Pratt, 2012). Many apps are free to users and companies providing free or purchased apps ultimately gain from selling ads within apps to be integrated.

Recent statistics (Mikulic, 2020) show the estimated size of the mobile medical apps market worldwide in 2017 in the total global market was valued at around 2.4 billion U.S. dollars and estimated to grow to over 11 billion dollars by 2025. Apple App store reported that the number of available medical apps there were 45,478 iOS healthcare apps available in 2019. the number of health apps being used by patients familiar to patients' groups being surveyed to manage their condition shows that more than 50 percent of patients familiar to surveyed patient groups used 1 or 2 health apps to manage their condition. More than 50 percent of patients used phone-based apps and more than 30 percent of the patients used web-based apps.

The most attractive healthcare sectors for mHealth app companies as of 2017, conducted among mHealth app developers included 30 percent of respondents named both "connection to doctors" and "diabetes" as the leading healthcare sectors for doing mHealth-connected business.

Australian sources report for example, OpenmHealth, that anyone can attempt to develop digital health tools, by taking advantage of open source resources for developers. Established businesses which are members of industry organizations (for example the Medical Software Industry Association; https://www.msia .com.au) are able to offer a grounded perspective on the viability of what you plan to develop as part of your digital health research and provide and get advisory services from professional and provider organization, such as: Pharmacy Guild of Australia Pharmacy innovations in digital health (eHealth). These forums provide information tools and methods that make valid data, information and knowledge resources available to consumers, and aims to understand and improve the ways that these tools or methods work, for example: to enable health access materially and intellectually by consumers; to address the health needs, interests and contexts of consumers; to allow consumers to interact directly with resources without a healthcare professional's facilitation in order to provide a personal and social framework that encompasses consumers' needs regarding their health needs and interests. These consumers' can improve their self-management and self-monitoring of health care plans and hence deepen consumers' engagement in clinical diagnosis, treatment and research.

When consumers download apps onto their smartphones or on social networking sites, their engagement with the apps provides marketers with useful insight into consumer behavior which means they've actively sought out the tools and features.

However, studies shows how sensitive data from health apps is finding its way to corporations with innovations in mobile personal computing, robotics, genomics, artificial intelligence promising to improve the quality, cost effectiveness, inclusivity, and patient care. Grundy and colleagues (2020) for example used an "app store crawling program" to identify the top 100 medicines related apps available to Android mobile users in the UK, USA, Australia, and Canada, combined with a search for endorsed apps on a medicines related agency website, a health app library, a systematic review, and their personal networks. Of the 821 apps screened, 24 met the criteria of managing drugs (for example, information, decision support, adherence, engagement) requesting at least one "dangerous" permission, claiming to collect or share user data, or requiring user interaction. Indeed, placing too much emphasis on autonomy and allowing individuals to take healthcare into their own hands can backfire. Commercial technologies have a low level of accountability because their aim is to lower costs. This is why principles addressing health needs as universal have been introduced and applied more than those addressing individual needs. Universal principles define patients as similar rather than as individuals with specific needs, skills or even preferences. This has led to the deep understanding among academics and health institutions that digital health should not be compatible with 'business as usual'; at levels from whole of clinic to whole of health system and whole of health profession, the effects are expected to be transformative or disruptive (Mano, 2019) pointing to the shadow of privacy risks.

CHAPTER 5

Health Systems

Health systems have addressed the new role of individuals as patient-consumers as a positive sign because they aimed to increase individuals' potential to enjoy better health. This positive approach aimed to alleviate the heavy costs of the traditional healthcare budgets and the development of concrete plans and strategies reflecting the social conditions and the potential of contact with (a) a health agent/provider (b) a health physical/virtual social setting. The first includes mostly the direct contact with a healthcare provider whereas the second reflects the influence of a larger health information locus such as the social media (Dutta-Bergman 2008). These macro level policies of the health systems and institutions encourage the development of digital services and programs that enable individuals to take more responsibility for their own health needs, diagnosis and treatment (Mano, 2019).

Analysis of health systems ranges from macro-level to micro-level perspectives. In other words, health systems seek to provide health answers to individuals as well as to whole populations by incorporating agents from the entire range of the health system. This may be why the *WHO Health Promotion Glossary* distinguishes between health promotion and other health concepts, such as burden of disease, capacity building, evidence-based health promotion, global health, health impact assessment, needs assessment, self-efficacy, social marketing, sustainable health promotion strategies, and wellness.

Healthcare systems are defined as the institutional entities responsible for providing health services and products to ensure the healthcare and wellbeing of the population. According to the World Health Organization, "a health system consists of all organizations." Indeed, today assessment of a health system includes both micro-level agents of health (*e.g.*, women and men caring for sick persons at home including children, disabled individuals and older members of the family), as well as macro-level agents (*e.g.*, health staff and other private providers responsible for health behavioral change programs, health insurance organizations and health and safety legislation). The literature addressing the importance of health systems focuses mainly on the different ways the government supplies the public with services and products that ensure solutions to individual health concerns.

A basic distinction in analyzing health systems is between two major types of health care systems—public and private. Additional typologies reflect the centrality of different criteria. The OECD concept is based on a combination of modes of governance and healthcare system characteristics, such as degree of coverage. This concept organizes healthcare arrangements along the following three dimensions: (1) access to healthcare as measured by the degree of population coverage; (2) sources of financing, such as general taxation, social insurance or private insurance; and (3) the public-private mix of healthcare provision.

Health system analysis takes into consideration the interrelations between public and private stakeholders who seek to introduce, advance and reform health. These interrelations may include multiple aspects, both at the level of individual healthcare as well as at the macro level of research and introduction of new health procedures and the mezzo level of management of within-sector relationships between healthcare professionals as the ones who promote health staff education and labor relations. The synergy between these is central to ensuring appropriate levels and quality of health services (Tollen, 2008). Indeed, health is now defined as the outcome of the complex interaction between multiple stakeholders. The ecological models that are widely used in the public health discourse stress the importance of a multilevel focus for health promotion (Sallis *et al.*, 2008; Winett, 1995). As a result the inclusion of various aspects of inter-sectoral action has been established, combining different institutional agents, such as the Ministry of Education to promote education for women and the Ministry of Welfare, to encourage individuals to study new as well as traditional health professions.

Scheiber (1987) pointed to three basic healthcare arrangements: (1) a national health service model with universal coverage, tax funding and public ownership of healthcare provision (*e.g.*, Sweden, Great Britain); (2) a social insurance model with universal coverage, social insurance financing and public or private ownership of facilities for healthcare provision (*e.g.*, Germany); and (3) a private insurance model with private coverage, financing and ownership of healthcare provision (*e.g.*, the United States) (Wendt, 2009). Other typologies focus on the different modes of governance and consider the role of political actors in the healthcare sector (Tuohy, 1999; Moran, 1999; Burau & Blank, 2006; Wendt *et al.*, 2009; Marmor & Wendt, 2011).

MICRO-LEVEL OUTCOMES OF HEALTH ASSESSMENT

Micro-level "subjective outcomes" can be measured and compared by describing how healthcare arrangements are understood by the population. This aspect is often expressed through the use of online health services (see *e.g.*, Mccoll-Kennedy *et al.*, 2017; Tian *et al.*, 2014). Indeed, individual behavior is the result of factors related to the level of expected services. If the level of expected service is high, the minimum level of expected service is also high and the range of tolerance is narrow. Some researchers who have examined how individuals use online health services (Kontos *et al.*, 2014; Kim *et al.*, 2012) suggest that the level of acceptance of online health services depends on the following factors:

- *Awareness of alternative services* that can affect the minimum level of expected services. If consumers have more alternatives, they set a higher minimum level of expectations than if fewer options are available.

- *Consumers' perceived role* in the provision and delivery of health services, which often depends on service quality. For example, when consumers are aware of their failure to comply with certain indications or treatments, their level of accepted service is lower.

- *Situational factors* (*e.g.*, emergency situations) can temporarily lower the minimum level of expectations. For example, an urgent dental problem may cause a consumer to seek out the nearest dentist.

- *Health literacy* is also associated with higher use of healthcare services, especially more specialized services.

- *Emergency situations* tend to raise the level of accepted service, for example when consumers waiting for a prompt response from their family doctor are not willing to wait any longer.

In line with this consumer and marketing approach, recent studies have begun to examine the use of online health services in terms of consumer behavior (Stefanscu *et al.*, 2019). According to the consumer approach, the provision of online health services must consider two basic components—threats and vulnerabilities in managing telehealth services. Stefanscu *et al.* (2019) suggest that online health service consumers are closely related to the providers of these services. Consumers are affected by providers' decisions, which often require agreements between different stakeholders representing various elements of service provision and its outcomes (Feng & Xie, 2015). Today, major investments are being directed toward the development and introduction of advanced health services and programs.

The effectiveness of online health services depends primarily on their accessibility and relevance, especially for self-management of health (Mano,

2019). This is why the process of providing outputs and outcomes in the health sector is based on complex integration of human- and technology-based elements, pointing to the constant need to evaluate online as well as offline services while considering several parameters, such as planning and tailoring (Cozica, 2014). For this reason, the differences between micro "subjective" measures and macro "objective" measures often become quite blurred due to a lesser focus on general health concerns caused by overemphasis on program efficiency. This issue becomes especially problematic when we consider the need to assess the impact of eHealth and mHealth access and the outcomes of health behaviors based upon variations in socio-demographic profiles and cultural effects. This is why according to Stokols (1992, 1996), the social, physical and cultural aspects of an environment have a cumulative effect on health.

The environment is a multilayered framework that affects individuals since institutions and neighborhoods are embedded in larger social and economic structures, and that the environmental context may influence the health of individual people differently, depending on their unique beliefs and practices. The above provides a partial explanation of why health institutions, HMOs and hospitals seek to maintain close contact with the recipients of their services by means of online health services (Stefanscu *et al.*, 2019). Through this approach, they are able to maintain contact with all target groups, including various institutions and organizations worldwide.

The major criteria for online health services include ease in using websites and the ability to book online appointments, obtain laboratory results, find a doctor and determine the strong points of the services offered (Stefanscu *et al.*, 2019; Zheng *et al.*, 2017). To this end, health systems and institutions encourage the development of services and programs that enable individuals to take more responsibility for their own health needs, diagnosis and treatment (Gurak & Hudson, 2006). Recent developments led to the creation of different types of people services online to enhance their well-being. In addition to providing informational value such as knowledge, these self-services offer instrumental value that seeks to increase health empowerment and use eHealth principles (see Kelson *et al.*, 2017; Stellefson *et al.*, 2011).

Consequently, an integrative approach is required. Such an approach should include the overall resources necessary for organizational performance, among them information resources, organizational resources, physical resources, human resources, and fiscal resources. These elements work together to determine how systems approach their relationships with other public and private agents in the area of health and more. According to Reichel *et al.*, (2019), comparisons between health systems should ultimately promote decision-making among policymakers, thus strengthening both political and social systems (Mossialos,1998; Jaeger, 2007).

IMACRO-LEVEL PERFORMANCE CRITERIA FOR HEALTH IMPACT ASSESSMENT

Efficiency in health expenditures has now become a central criterion in assessing the performance of health systems that seek to relieve the pressure of expenditures generated by the growing numbers of aging individuals (Heller & Hauner, 2006) and their associated healthcare needs. Nevertheless, the concepts use by the various stakeholders are so diverse that it is difficult to integrate them within a single message or post.

Health impact assessment entails a combination of procedures, methods and tools by which a policy, program, product, or service may be judged with respect to its effects on the health of the population (WHO Regional Office for Europe, 1999). According to Wendt and Kohl (2010), comparisons between health systems find expression in the ways that countries with a higher share of public health expenditures effectively control their healthcare costs. A comprehensive way to measure the effectiveness and efficiency of health systems can be derived by bearing in mind that health impact assessment considers both positive and negative effects and can be used to identify new opportunities for health promotion (Smith *et al.*, 2006; Kearney *et al.*, 2019) and promoted the importance of "likes" in HPV vaccination (Miller *et al.*, 2019). Similarly, in the study of health in terms of networks, Barker and Rohde (2019) emphasized the efficiency of online communities in smoking prevention. More and more studies (Bekalu *et al.*, 2019) confirm that social media should be integrated into users' social routines for issues related to preventive health practices (Evans *et al.*, 2019; Johnson *et al.*, 2019). In order to do so, an analysis of different systems necessitates referring to and examining three different levels of health systems is necessary.

First, it is important to examine how societies move from a societal level of healthcare to a public system. Second, it is essential to identify how the system changes from within when the interrelations between the actors change. And finally, it is critical to discover whether and to what extent imposed regulation changes transform the carriers of services and products (Wendt *et al.*, 2009, p. 83), facilitating a careful combination of policy and identified problems (Kutzin *et al.*, 2010, p. 384). These distinctions have been partly adopted in developing countries as well. In particular, developing nations with large rural areas and populations have more crucial healthcare issues to deal with, such as the prevalence of chronic infectious diseases, the lack of adequately trained healthcare personnel and healthcare facilities, and the limited number of healthcare programs (World Health Organization, 2006).

The European Observatory on Health Systems and Policies (HiTs) focuses on how a health system is organized, how funds flow through the system, and what care it provides (Reichel *et al.*, 2019), while considering the variations emerging when health impact assessment is conducted at the local or regional level. Nevertheless, the literature addressing the importance of health systems focuses mainly on the different ways states supply services and products to the public that ensure solutions to individual health concerns. Only recently have typologies begun to focus on micro-level variations among individuals and on patient access to healthcare (Wendt, 2009; Reibling, 2010).

Indeed, recent studies emphasize the importance of addressing health issues with a stakeholder approach to health. The efficiency of health systems is therefore evaluated by both subjective (reported user satisfaction) and objective (level of health expenditures) terms. Reibling (2010) placed even more emphasis on patient access to healthcare services, using the criteria of gatekeeping, cost-sharing, provider density (GPs, specialists, and nurses) and medical technology (magnetic resonance imaging units/MRI, computed tomography scanners/CT). These patient-centered typologies make it possible to assess relationships among healthcare systems, access to healthcare services, and health outcomes. Yet implementing this type of total stakeholder approach is more often than not elusive for the health organizations making up the health systems. Moreover, these tendencies have become more complex with the introduction of eHealth and mHealth technologies. Access to services facilitates an effective combination between the needs of individuals and those of health care organizations (Smith & Busse, 2009).

Measuring patient utilization of healthcare services is another way to analyze outcome variations in different countries. The association between utilization differences among socio-economic groups and healthcare features has been extensively investigated in the equity literature, especially the work of van Doorslaer and Masuria (2004). These studies pointed to differences in healthcare utilization related to income variations, such that individuals with low incomes use medical services more frequently. Similarly, Van Doorslaer Masseria and Koolman (2006) showed that visits to physicians are also more prevalent among poorer groups than among well-to-do individuals. This tendency has been assessed in cross-sectional studies in nearly every country. The authors concluded that inequity reflects patient-initiated attitudes and behaviors and less those of physicians.

In some studies (Reibling & Wendt, 2011), concerns are raised regarding the way formal regulation of patient access to healthcare should be undertaken through a gatekeeping system that addresses differences in healthcare utilization between income and educational groups. They found that the intensity of regulation affects healthcare utilization differently for different educational levels. While these differences were mostly evident in visits to specialists, they clearly indicate that measuring healthcare system performance (Smith *et al.*, 2009) necessitates considering the impact of multiple factors at both the micro-and macro-levels that address issues of health status, clinical quality and appropriateness of care, healthcare system responsiveness, equity and productivity (Smith *et al.*, 2012).

INSTITUTIONAL USE OF SOCIAL MEDIA

Healthcare institutions encourage active use of social media to raise health awareness, distribute information, engage stakeholders, or drive traffic to their main websites (Park, Rodgers & Stemmle, 2011; Korda & Itani, 2013; Zhang, 2013). Social media also serve as a platform for interaction between users on health issues (Li, 2013; Newman *et al.*, 2011) to improve healthcare behavior and communication (Erbes *et al.*, 2014; Miller *et al.*, 2016).

Health portals play a central role in the use of digital technology for health purposes. The recently observed increase in the use of patient portals emphasizes the importance of patient engagement. When people engage in social exchange, they talk to each more frequently to exchange information or opinions. Deng *et al.*, (2019) report for example that user satisfaction with health portals exerted a positive impact on intentions to continue using these services. According to the social contagion theory, behaviors are subject to the opinions of people who are important to a particular individual (Christakis & Fowler, 2013; Heath & Porter, 2017). Portal users with more positive input about portals from their close social circle are themselves more likely to be satisfied with the portal. Oghuma *et al.* (2016) demonstrated how perceived service quality and perceived usability can affect satisfaction, which in turn influences use continuance.

This finding calls for a thorough evaluation of the quality of these portals. Allegrante and Auld (2019) indicate that understanding the effectiveness of social media for health purposes necessitates first understanding the extent to which users are satisfied with the overall effects of technology in their lives. Indeed, more frequent delivery of messages to priority populations in public health can promote health behavior changes (Mano, 2019). One such example is sending messages about the risks of hookah tobacco use to young adult hookah smokers (Johnson *et al.* 2019). Similarly, de los Reyes (2019) highlights the challenges and opportunities facing institutional entrepreneurship in digital public health

(Tang *et al.*, 2019). Indeed, recent studies (Riley *et al.*, 2019) conclude that research of mHealth necessitates considering both the challenges and opportunities in the digital health field. Institutional health providers continued to emphasize the role of individuals as patient-consumers as a positive sign that individuals will be able to enjoy better health. At the same time, this will alleviate the heavy costs of traditional healthcare budgets, especially in view of the constant increase in virtual sources of health and mobile applications used by institutional healthcare providers to improve health services. Yet institutional healthcare providers are also challenged by this "information control" process because patients may challenge the authority of their health provider, especially those facing difficult health conditions. More importantly, the possibility of permitting people to use technology independently for health purposes remains up for discussion because many factors influence the use and abandonment of these technologies including accessibility, experience and usability (Antona & Stephanidis, 2020).

Despite the important steps taken in these three such as reducing the amount of information to be transmitted, avoiding unnecessary actions and elements for the application, prioritizing the mobile layout, reducing the effort and time spent, and providing a pleasant experience are all important factors yet often gone missing due to a higher focus on technological efficiency. For this reason, it remains important to continue examining individuals' routine use of social media relative to their feelings about the significance of social media and technology for health so as to reduce possible negative feelings about social media use (Ellison *et al.*, 2007; Steinfield *et al.*, 2008), especially in the context of issues of trust and privacy violations (Tang *et al.*, 2019; Adams, 2010).

CHAPTER 6

The COVID-19 Pandemic and Digital Divides

The advantages of the internet as a source of health information include convenient access to a massive volume of information, ease of updating information and interactive formats that promote understanding and retention of information. The health empowerment paradigm has introduced the notion of health efficacy and the right to express health aspirations, thus enabling individuals to develop critical awareness about their existing health conditions (Bandura, 1977; Bandura, 2004; Dutta-Bergman, 2006). These models rely on two assumptions: First, as noted, easy access to information will give rise to rational consumer choice, such that individuals will be motivated to seek even more information and compare between multiple sources of information before making health decisions (Dutta-Bergman, 2006). Second, all individuals are equally able to learn and internalize aspects of health and disease. Hence, these models assess the functional aspects of digital technology and the way they complement each (Mesch *et al.*, 2012).

THE NORMALIZATION HYPOTHESIS

According to the normalization hypothesis, the rise of the information society and the adoption of the internet have the capacity to reduce existing social inequalities in health. The prominence of the normalization hypothesis suggests that technology will ultimately minimize differences between individuals characterized by different socioeconomic variations such as education, income, occupation, gender and ethnicity (Hargitai & Hinnant, 2008; Lemire, *et al.*, 2008; Renahy *et al.*, 2008). Indeed, studies in the field of communication have pursued this line of thought. More specifically, the Media-System Dependency theory suggests that resources located on the internet allow users to explore a health topic fully. Users can also use the internet as a communications tool to increase their capacity to attain their goals, such as changing health behavior, engaging in physical activity and/or ceasing smoking (Dutta-Bergman, 2006; 2004b).

THE SOCIAL DIVERSIFICATION HYPOTHESIS

According to the social diversification hypothesis, computer-mediated communication provides a platform for overcoming social inequalities in access to information and social networks. Residential and social segregation prevents members of minority groups from interacting across ethnicity and migration status (Mesch *et al.*, 2012). Consequently, segregation reduces access to social networks that have the potential to provide available information on health-related conditions. Studies examining differences in access to health information in the US found a high level of agreement among African-Americans and Hispanics that the internet is a helpful resource for health information. There is both motivation and need for accessing health information, in particular among low income members of minority groups. Accordingly, the social diversification perspective maintains that disadvantaged groups (due to migration status and ethnicity) will use the internet to expand their social circles, to diversify their sources of information and social networks through computer-mediated communication and to access non-redundant information and networks. At the same time, majority groups will use ICT to maintain their existing levels of information and social networks, for example through interpersonal communication and direct communication with health providers. Indeed, some individuals or even entire groups of people are less likely to express health-related aspirations and expectations or to develop health-related consciousness.

The concept of a digital divide indeed reflects inequalities in access and use of online information and services and unequal outcomes in health. In turn, the outcome of ICT access and use may affect the motivations and beliefs of social groups, as shown in early studies of internet uses and outcomes (Van Dijk, 2006). Generally, this literature found that digital inequalities tend to mirror existing social inequalities in terms of socioeconomic status, education, gender, age, geographic location, employment status, and race (Robinson *et al.*, 2015).

FIRST LEVEL DIGITAL DIVIDE EFFECTS

Differences in access to technology are also called first-level digital divides (Wyatt *et al.*, 2000; Gui & Argentin, 2011). In contrast to the functional approach, demographic and socioeconomic factors (Lemire, *et al.*, 2008; Renahy *et al.*, 2008) and health status (Mano, 2016, 2018) play an important role in defining the depth of the first digital divide. Kolasa *et al.* (2020) for example, showed that sociodemographic factors influence the use of e-health among individuals with chronic conditions, and Fabienne Reiners *et al.* (2019) indicated that e-health seems to be used the least by those that may need it the most, such as older individuals and those with chronic diseases, low incomes and low educational levels who live in rural areas. Indeed, the use of virtual devices can initiate first-level digital divide effects on access to health-related information. The already disadvantaged citizens in society are equally disadvantaged on the internet, either through their limited access to technology and restricted opportunities for use, and / or lack of important digital skills (Hargittai, 2002; Hargittai & Hinnant, 2008; Robinson, 2009; Sims, 2014; Zillien & Hargittai, 2009). Such groups will be less likely to capitalize on information technology than more privileged groups (Blank & Lutz, 2018; Van Deursen & Helsper, 2015).

Age

Due to age's high correlation with technology and internet skills, elderly people are less likely to know how to use the internet and search engines and less likely to use these extensively (Van Deursen *et al.*, 2010). Since health usually deteriorates with age (Hardt & Hollis-Sawyer, 2007), growing older provides an important motivation for seeking online health-related information and participating in group discussions about health (Bundorf *et al.*, 2006). Recent studies also consistently point to the negative effect of age on health-related use of social media (Thackeray *et al.*, 2013). Older users tend to adopt technology later and are less internet savvy than younger users (Mesch, 2012). In fact, individuals who are 50-60 years old tend to search mainly for health information, while individuals who are between 60-80 years old search less due to the lack of computer skills. Moreover, because older people are more likely to be affected by health-related issues, differences in age are likely to be significant. Since health tends to deteriorate with age (Mano, 2016), older users are also less able to learn and become adept at health-related social media use. Therefore, they are also less likely to be influenced by health information on social media than younger users. Indeed, the 'grey divide' (Morris & Brading, 2007) continues to be documented in various internet studies (Demunter, 2005; Katz & Rice, 2002; Latzer *et al.*, 2013; Loges & Jung, 2001; Smith, 2014; Wei, 2012), possibly because the age barriers of trust are greater than any technological barriers.

Evidence points to age differences between older and younger adults in trust placed in health information on the internet. Younger adults appear to be more inclined to use the internet for health information regardless of their trust in this information, and this use can have a positive effect on their health behaviors (Fox & Rainie, 2000; Shim *et al.*, 2006). Many older adults who could go online to expand their knowledge of disease management, treatment options, and diet and exercise are not doing so (Hart *et al.*, 2004). Thus, the full potential of the internet in supporting healthy aging is not being realized. In light of research showing that knowledge is an important predictor of online health searches (Hong, 2006) and search effectiveness (Keselman *et al.*, 2008), helping older adults overcome barriers to searching for health information online is of great importance. Over time, successful searches have the potential to support gains in health literacy and slow the effects of age on cognition by helping older adults rely more on knowledge (declarative and procedural) and less on age-sensitive cognitive abilities (Miller, 2010; Miller *et al.*, 2011; Miller *et al.*, 2010).

Health Status

State of illness is almost always related to online health information search and health behavior changes (Dutta-Bergman, 2006). *Chronic disease* significantly increases the likelihood that a user will work on a blog or contribute to an online discussion, a listserv or some other online group or forum that helps people with personal issues or health problems. Specific health conditions motivate individuals to begin searching online to retrieve relevant information. In fact such differences in health status limit access and use of online health information are reduce the individuals' potential for health empowerment (Rice, 2006; Sciamanna *et al.*, 2004) and wellbeing, including health self-management (HM) and social resilience (HR) among aging individuals (Rice, 2006; Sciamanna *et al.*, 2004), and to contribute to the notion of "healthy" aging (Bowling & Dieppe, 2005). Since patients, healthcare organizations and public service agencies have begun relying more and more on the internet as a channel for providing services (Andreassen *et al.*, 2007), differences may emerge between individuals with various chronic conditions, especially when these differences stem from educational gaps. Existing evidence indicates that individuals with chronic health conditions who have lower educational levels will be less able to find the information they seek than those with similar health concerns who are more educated (Manhattan Research, 2012).

Gender

Gender is an important factor in online behavior. Women tend to search for health information on all media (Rice, 2006) more than men, and these differences are apparent in the use of online medical information as well (Renahy *et al.*, 2008; Cotten & Gupta, 2004; Lorence, *et al.*, 2006). Men tend to use online information more than women to ask physicians questions, whereas women use online information more to inform family members. According to the Pew Internet Project (2008), women are more likely than men to turn to the internet for diagnoses. Indeed, 35% of women went online specifically to find out about a medical condition for themselves or someone else (Ybarra & Suman, 2008). Recent studies of gender differences in searching for health information online

(Chen & Lee, 2014; Mesch *et al.*, 2012; Yan, 2010) indicate that the apparent reason women search for health information more than men is their traditional role as caregivers (Mano, 2016) and socialization processes developed during early childhood. Wilhelm and Bekkers (2010) refer to this as the principle of care, a side-effect of compassion.

Education

The advantages of the internet as a source of health information include convenient access to a massive volume of information, ease in updating information, and interactive formats that promote understanding and retention of information. Higher education levels reflect greater motivation to engage in healthier behaviors (Chew *et al.*, 1998), search for health information (Mesch *et al.*, 2012) and consult online health-related rankings and reviews (Thackeray *et al.*, 2013). Therefore, individuals with academic education are also more likely to be influenced by health information on social media than those with lower levels of education (Mano, 2019; Rosenberg *et al.*, 2020). Based on this notion of a first-level digital divide, it is also important to recognize how differences in digital skills create new inequalities, generating a second-level digital divide (Gui & Argentin, 2011; Hargittai, 2002; van Deursen & van Dijk, 2010; Dobson & Willinsky, 2009; Eshet & Aviram, 2006; Eshet-Alkalai & Chajut, 2009; Hargittai, 2005, 2009; Jenkins *et al.*, 2006; Livingstone & Helsper, 2010; Perez-Tornero, 2004).

SECOND-LEVEL DIGITAL DIVIDE

The second-level digital divide extends the notion of the first-level digital divide beyond access to issues related to health services. In contrast to the health empowerment perspective, the notion of a secondary digital divide suggests that more and more aspects of individual and group behaviors are affected by differences in access to and use of online services (Hargittai, 2010; Hargittai & Hinnant, 2008; Van Deursen & Van Dijk, 2011, 2014; Van Dijk, 2006; Zillien & Hargittai, 2009). These studies point to inequalities in how often individuals perform different types of online behavior and differentiate active content creators from passive consumers and identify user characteristics for specific social media platforms (*e.g.*, Blank, 2013; Blank & Lutz, 2017; Brake, 2014; Correa, 2010; Hargittai, 2007, 2015; Hargittai & Walejko, 2008; Hoffmann *et al.*, 2015; Schradie, 2011). Considering that the strong associations between socioeconomic status and online participation or social media use (Lutz, 2016) may not be reliable, most studies show that age remains a strong predictor of online participation and social media use and the gender influences types of health-related behavior and other platforms (Pew, 2018b). Moreover, the second-level digital divide has also been shown to be related to online activities for recreational purposes and work (Mano, 2019).

Technology Skills

Differences between adoption, access and more specific usage patterns and skills constitute a pivotal breakthrough in analyzing the impact of technology skills on the use of digital sources of health (Pearce & Rice, 2013). Adoption differentiates between those who have and those who have not used the internet, whereas usage reveals the level of dependency on online sources, including those related to health. After internet access has been achieved, skills and literacy become important because more use signifies greater skills and more literacy. For this reason, discrepancies in skills and literacy have become known as the second-level digital divide (Dewan and Riggins, 2005; Mossberger *et al*., 2003; Van Deursen & Van Dijk, 2011).

Indeed, variations in technology skills are important outcomes of the first-level digital divide. Internet access has approached saturation in most affluent societies. Nevertheless, a specialized look at internet use points to variations. Lee *et al*. (2011) identify four factors that influence internet usage among older adults: (1) intrapersonal factors such as motivation and self-efficacy, (2) functional limitations such as decline of memory or spatial orientation, (3) structural limitations such as costs, and (4) interpersonal limitations such as the lack of encouragement to begin using the internet or no one to send an email to. These variations result in differentiating older adults into three age groups: pre-seniors (ages 50–64), young-olds (ages 65–74) and old-olds (age 75+). Due to the relationship between age and cognitive strength, each one of these three age groups may respond differently to similar digital stimuli, with the younger groups more motivated to try novel ways of using health applications and online services (Mano, 2021). Success can be achieved by promoting adoption of platforms that rely more on basic audio-visual skills and less on education-sensitive cognitive abilities (Miller *et al*., 2011; Miller *et al*., 2010).

THIRD LEVEL DIGITAL DIVIDE EFFECTS

Third-level divides relate to gaps in individuals' capacity to translate their internet access and use into favorable outcomes (Van Deursen & Helsper, 2015, p. 30). These discrepancies are also related to the increase in mobile devices, indicating that the digital divide is expanding with the growth of the mobile internet (Marler, 2018; Pearce & Rice, 2013) and other mobile technologies (Van der Zeeuw *et al*.,

2019). These trends have been confirmed in many countries, including the United States (Hargittai & Hinnant, 2008), where around 90% of the population has access to the internet (Pew, 2018a), and globally (International Telecommunications Union, 2017), particularly among individuals living in rural areas, those aged 65+, and those with less than a high school degree (Pew, 2018a). Moreover, Napoli and Obar (2014) suggested therefor that a mobile internet "underclass" has been created that manifests in problems associated with mobile internet access. Internet access through mobile technology has a lower potential for speedy access and storage, and limitations due to screen size and keyboard use may become a problem in undertaking daily tasks, such as editing text documents and tables (Tsetsi & Rains, 2017), that are often necessary to increase work effectiveness and reduce anxieties (Mano & Mesch, 2010).

International Comparisons

A major perspective addressing the notion of third-level divides emerges in the cultural perspective that indicates that ethnocentric patterns of health information preference remained relatively stable at different educational levels, implying that the effect of patients' ethnicity influenced information preference more than education. individuals in more traditional cultural settings (Kvasny, 2006) as opposed to modern cultures (Lutz, 2016), are more likely to feel confident about using technology (Zainuddin *et al.*, 2016). This leads to differences in self-efficacy either in using technology for accessing information and/or in the ability to be part of an online service process. Among these individuals and groups, the likelihood of participating in a provider/customer service production process is low, while adhering to traditional human relationships remains a strong preference (Gümüş & Sönmez, 2020; Anderson & Ostrom, 2015; Ostrom *et al.*, 2015; Zhang *et al.*, 2017; Mano, 2016; Scheerder *et al.*, 2017). As a result, the expected technology-driven empowerment in health may not take place if improvements are not made in the necessary skills and attitudes to account for cultural variations in the use of online health (see *e.g.*, Mccoll-Kennedy *et al.*, 2017; Tian *et al.*, 2014). They suggested that these differences highlighted the importance of recognizing culturally developed world views when understanding their health information seeking behavior (Rosenberg *et al.*, 2019).

Ethnic affiliation is a central factor when immigrants face barriers in internet access and use. According to the communication infrastructure theory, ethnic communities differ in their communication opportunity structures. Some environments afford easy connections to necessary and useful communication channels, but others make it difficult to access communication channels. Differences in communication opportunity structures are the result of social stratification processes and are associated with differential access to social, political, cultural and social capital resources. Whether such disparities are fully explained by socioeconomic factors or whether they constitute a unique cultural effect that remains after socioeconomic factors are controlled is unclear.

Some studies show that the internet has become integrated into the communication infrastructure of white neighborhoods but less so in immigrant neighborhoods. Similarly, studies on differences in access to health information in the US found a high level of agreement among African-Americans and Hispanics that the internet is a helpful resource for health information, in particular for people with low incomes, older persons or those disabled due to illness (Lorence *et al.*, 2006). This has created a magnifying glass effect, for those who need to compensate for lack of social capital by expanding their social networks and access new information in Israel among Arab and Jewish residential areas as well (Rosenberg *et al.*, 2019). Hence, it is possible to assume that the gaps between these groups and the "privileged" ones are reflected in level of access and understanding of health information.

Ethnic gaps may serve to increase social inequalities in health care and ultimately create differences in the level of health quality between minorities and the majority group (Arie & Mesch, 2015; Gonzalez, 2017; Mesch, 2012; Mesch *et al.*, 2012). In an earlier study (Kakai *et al.*, 2003), disparities in access to information between Asian and Caucasian cancer patients were found in Hawaii and three clusters of health information were revealed to be related to three ethnic groups: Caucasian, Japanese, and Asian non-Japanese. The results of this study revealed that Caucasian patients preferred objective, scientific, and updated information obtained through medical journals or newsletters from research institutions, telephone information services, and the Internet. Japanese patients relied on media and commercial sources, including television, newspapers, books, magazines, and CAM providers. Non-Japanese Asians and Pacific Islanders used information sources involving person-to-person communication with their physicians, social groups, and other cancer patients. Higher educational levels were observed relative to preferences for health information that emphasized objective, scientific, and updated information, while lower education was associated with personally communicated information.

The low-cost equipment of infrastructure and the prepaid technology make millions of people in the world, especially in the developing countries to be able to afford mobile phones (Kalba, 2008b). Many scholars conducted research to explore the rapid mobile phone diffusion in developing countries. For example, Loo and Ngan (2012) and Lim *et al.* (2015) demonstrated that China implemented successful strategies to diffuse mobile phone, and now become the biggest mobile market in the world. Srinuan *et al.* (2012) investigated how mobile phones had been rapidly adopted in Thailand. Their study showed that the adoption rate of mobile phones of Thailand in 2003 was 33%, and this rate already exceeded 100% in 2010. There are many other similar studies on other countries, such as India, Vietnam, Peru, *etc.* (Hwang *et al.*, 2009; Gupta & Jain, 2012; Yamakawa *et al.*, 2013). And many of these studies stated that mobile phone has become an access platform to the Internet, and hence bridged the digital divide between developed countries and developing countries (Loo & Ngan, 2012; Kalba, 2008b; Mir and Dangerfield, 2013; Prieger, 2013; Srinuan *et al.*, 2012).

Nonetheless, the cultural perspective goes beyond the uses and gratifications theory, suggesting the individuals use technology to satisfy their needs. When people use media for specific purposes, they seek the added value provided by the information they need to accomplish specific tasks (see *e.g.*, Dholakia *et al.*, 2004). The perceived usefulness determine acceptability manifest in willingness to participate in online processes concerning health. This process is evident among individuals with different cultural backgrounds (Rosenberg *et al.*, 2019). This is also true for topics related to health especially when these are related to the use of health support groups and buying health products and services (Barak & Grohol, 2011) as well as to enhancing health and well-being.

In fact, the concept of *affordances* refers to how individuals adapt to *technology*. Affordances capture the beneficial/injurious aspect of objects and are relative in terms of how well objects fit an individual situation. The strength of affordances lies in the individual's perceptions regarding the need to weigh one's "action possibilities" (Norman, 2002). In ICT studies, the term "affordances" denotes the need to address everyday objects together with their features and functions. It also suggests that when using a device, individuals may think more about the uses it "affords" than about its "objective" qualities. This is because ICT features and functions do not necessarily "fit" the needs of users. The lack of "fit" between personal affordance and ICT features reflects the impact of personal circumstances that may either encourage or discourage individuals from developing favorable ICT attitudes. This lack of fit generates a chain of health attitudes and behaviors.

CHAPTER 7

The Case of COVID-19 and Digital Divides

The global crisis caused by COVID-19 has changed the reality of individuals in many ways and brought new conditions of financial and social ambiguity. Individuals experienced a substantial loss of social and economic resources, which increased vulnerability and affected resilience. The complexity of a crisis such as COVD -19 can be better understood by focusing on the role of technology (Reghezza-Zitt & Rufat, 2019). In light of research showing that knowledge is an important predictor of online health searching and search effectiveness (Keselman *et al.*, 2008), we can expect that successful online searches and use of health forums will improve resilience in times of crisis such as the pandemic COVID-19.

Resilience is defined as the process of effectively negotiating, adapting to, or managing significant sources of stress or trauma. Individuals seeking to regain control of the situation are likely to use the resources not affected by the crisis to install stability (Masten, 2018; Vindevogel, 2017). Resilience studies focus on positive recovery and adaptation processes and the analysis of a system's strengths, resilience has been gradually associated with social-ecological factors important in developing the sense of well-being under stress (Ungar, 2011b). Resilience in the COVID-19 crisis, according to the American Psychological Association, is the process of adequate adaptation to significant stressors and the potential for quick and decisive recovery, especially in times of crises when individuals need social support (Sippel *et al.*, 2015). In order for resilience to rake place rapidly and completely resources should be available and accessible immediately. These resources should be abundant so that individuals would not compete be destroyed by excessive use. This is the case of social media use.

Online platforms of connectivity provide individuals with a platform that overcomes barriers of distance and time to connect and reconnect with others and thereby expand and strengthen their offline networks and interactions (Antoci *et al.*, 2015; Hall *et al.*, 2018; Subrahmanyam *et al.*, 2008; Twenge *et al.*, 2018).

Originally, social media has been regarded as an important source of information especially when individuals are in a state of uncertainty and possible dissatisfaction with existing sources of information (Ogawa, 2011; Jung & Moro,

2014; Chan, 2013) and hence lower discomfort (Wixom & Todd, 2005; Wang *et al.*, 2012; Rosenberg *et al.*, 2019) that is especially important in times of crisis (Chan, 2013) such as the pandemic COVID-19.

Indeed, social media is a significant resource that is abundant and can protect against the detrimental effects of stress and threat commonly experienced by individuals during crises and enhance experiences of well-being (Barasa *et al.*, 2018). Social media can therefore increase significantly the level of resilience among individuals who experience crises (Mano *et al.*, 2019). An influential model addressing resilience is that of Norris and colleagues (2008). The model addresses resilience in community as the outcome of networked resources including economic development, social capital, and information communication. Indeed, Chan maintains that "by harnessing the characteristics of the social media tools, organizational capacity to demonstrate resilience in response to crises can be significantly enhanced by creating new avenues for collaboration to help build more resilient communities over time" (Chan, 2013; p. 5; Whittaker *et al.*, 2015).

Witnessing now how online health services become an institutionalized form of service provision in the health industry it is important to identify the possible sources of deepening health digital divides (Mano, 2016; Marler, 2018), in order to increase the resilience of weak social groups (Robinson *et al.*, 2015). This is especially evident among those most in need of health empowerment—the elderly, those located in remote geographic areas, and/or those coping with chronic illnesses and disabilities (Hadwich *et al.*, 2006; Eisenberg & Berkowitz, 2009; Aceijas, 2011; Mano, 2016). More importantly, not all individuals develop the necessary levels of confidence that enable them to adhere to a healthier and focused approach (McKinley& Wright, 2014). Since all types of empowerment necessitate taking responsibility, asking questions and acting upon them (Fox *et al.*, 2005), it is not surprising that some individual-level factors are likely to affect the acquisition of greater health literacy and empowerment (Baran & Davis, 2009; Ginossar & Nelson 2010). As a result, while the internet can improve health empowerment and encourage successful self-management practices, evidence indicates that differences in the use of online services reflect differences in socioeconomic status (Lorence *et al*, 2006; Lemire *et al*, 2008; Renahy *et al.*, 2008). The concept of a third-level digital divide addresses differences in gains from internet use, particularly where access and use patterns are roughly similar. In the COVID-19, an important outcome of online forums is the potential to increase resilience (Notton, 2008).

POSITIVE EFFECTS ON RESILIENCE

First, social media decreases the likelihood of social isolation and increases the potential for virtual connectivity that facilitates the sense of belonging and togetherness (Maarten *et al.*, 2009; Valkenburg & Schouten, 2006). These in turn decrease loneliness (Burke *et al.*, 2010; Stepanikova *et al.*, 2010). Second, social media lowers discomfort because it increases the potential of expression that is often limited in day-to-day interactions (Wixom & Todd, 2005; Wang *et al.*, 2012; Rosenberg *et al.*, 2019) that is especially important in times of crisis (Chan, 2013). Third, social media increases the likelihood for positive social support from social groups, family, friendships and community (Davis, 2012; Dolev-Cohen & Barak, 2013; Diener, 2009; Helliwell & Wang, 2011; Huang, 2012) that are especially important when we are disconnected from the external environment (Marcopulos, 2009). The notion of social support is especially noticed because it mediates the effects of life stress on health and well-being (Pawar AA, Rathod 2007; Sippel *et al.*, 2015). Positive social support can provide protection against stress and facilitate in development of individual resilience among individuals who face significant adversity (Ungar, 2011; Zautra *et al.*, 2010). Fourth, social media use has been associated with a decrease in depression and loneliness and an increase in self-esteem and social support among this population (Shaw & Gant 2004). Finally, online activity can increase resilience as well. Social media includes a variety of online activities involving the use of profiles, comments, photos, or video sharing. These expand the depth and extent of connectivity (Kavanaugh *et al.*, 2005; Jurgens & Helsloot, 2018) and enable individuals to expand their network (Smith & Kidder, 2010) thus improving that chances for more extensive social support once the crisis is over. While social media use has been linked to psychological well-being, the findings have not been unanimous.

NEGATIVE EFFECTS ON RESILIENCE

The fact that social media use is considered to have become popular across all age groups (Smith & Anderson, 2018) is still debated especially because most studies have focused on adolescent and young adults in college settings (*e.g.*, Booker *et al.*, 2018; Ellison *et al.*, 2007; Kross *et al.*, 2013). The specific of these samples in terms of age led to a growing body of research asking how social media use is associated with some health-related outcomes. For example, a recent longitudinal study found that Facebook use is generally negatively associated with mental well-being (Shakya & Christakis, 2017). Another study examining the influence of Facebook use on subjective well-being over time among young adults found that Facebook, rather than enhancing well-being, might undermine it (Kross *et al.*, 2013). Several recent studies have also found negative associations of social media use with a variety of indicators of mental health among adolescents and young adults. For example, in a study drawing data from a sample of adolescents and their parents throughout the United States, Barry *et al.*, (2017) found that social media use is moderately and positively related to adolescent-reported fear of missing out and loneliness as well as with parent-reported hyperactivity/ impulsivity, anxiety, and depression.

Similarly, Berryman *et al.*, (2018) found that while overall social media use was not predictive of impaired mental health functioning, one particular activity, that is, "vaguebooking" (posting unclear but alarming posts to get attention), was found to be predictive of suicidal ideation among young adults. Another study that assessed the impact of overall social media use, night-time-specific social media use, and emotional investment in social media are more important than overall use in determining adolescent sleep and well-being (Woods & Scott, 2016).

SOCIAL MEDIA VARIATIONS EFFECTS ON RESILIENCE

Specific features of online platform may create variations in outcomes. Some platforms are based on written interaction (Twitter, Tumblr) are show to affect negatively resilience whereas other platforms such as Instagram, focusing on photo-sharing, was rather positively associated with positive mental health variables. (Zakour, 2019). Recent studies predict various aspects of users behaviour in the context of social media use (Wixom & Todd, 2005; Wang *et al.*, 2012). Rosenberg *et al.*, (2019) conclude that social media have become popular because they can fulfil users' various needs related to social connections through the perspective of uses and gratification theory (Katz *et al.*, 1973). On other cases, excessive use of these networks may have adverse effect on wellbeing mainly when information shares involves "misinformation". Brailovskaia and Margraf (2016) for example comparing Facebook users and non-users shows that while Facebook users had higher values of life satisfaction, happiness and social support, non-users showed higher depression symptoms. Other studies indicate how social media use can decrease real-life social interactions decreasing mental health and well-being (Berryman *et al.*, 2018; Hall *et al.*, 2018). Evidence also indicates that social media increases adolescents' depression symptoms (Rosen *et al.*, 2013; Ra *et al.*, 2018; Laura & Choate, 2017) causing high dissatisfaction and anxiety (Vogue & Mills, 2018; Booker *et al.*, 2018) and subjective well-being (Kim & Kim, 2017) to the point that for some individuals social media use appears to be meaningless (Sagioglu & Greitemeyer, 2014). In a national survey of U.S. young adults, Primack *et al.*, (2017) found that compared with individuals who use 0 to 2 social media platforms, individuals who use 7 to 11 social media platforms have substantially higher odds of having increased levels of depression and anxiety symptoms. In a recent study among U.S. adolescents, Ra *et al.*, (2018) have also found a statistically significant but modest association between higher frequency of digital media use and subsequent symptoms of attention-deficit/hyperactivity disorder. This is why Frison and Eggermont (2015) suggested a distinction between Facebook users and revealed that adolescents' well-being depending on type of use—whether it was "active" or "passive" use. According to this study, active Facebook use were more likely to report positive outcomes, relatively to the passive users who reported they did not actively engaged in exchanges and merely viewed others' posts.

These variations certainly can shape the potential to use online platforms and social media as a source of support and access to resources. Since variations in technology use and internet access are frequently related to socioeconomic status differences the potential of having access to the abundance of information and services is reduced and hence lower the potential for access to deliveries, necessary for the normal attendance to everyday tasks such as cooking, schooling devices providing educational frameworks for younger, medical attendance and connectivity for older family members and work-related procedures such as ZOOM necessary for the completion of tasks and connecting with work settings (Ifinedo, 2016). This is why we need to assess how routine *versus* occasional use of social media use may have differential effects on wellness and resilience (Meslin *et al.*, 2019) during the COVID-19.

CHAPTER 8

Discussion

The shift from "mechanical" to "informational" medicine has placed responsibility for health on individuals and on their ability to increase their own health awareness, particularly through personal involvement and access to health information. For many of us, this means that our social profile has expanded over time due to easy and cheap access to information, people and online communities. Everyday activities such as communicating with others, purchasing goods, banking, and searching for any kind of information have now become easier and more accessible. These changes have led to the development and introduction of a significant number of online health resources. Over time, individuals have become technologically skilled and willing to access sources of health-related information, participate in networking sites and search the web. Indeed, accessing the information we seek either on our own or with unsolicited support from online health forums as well as participation in support groups providing medical advice and online services may be too easy. Institutional healthcare providers emphasize low costs and efficient provision of health literacy through various forms of virtual connectivity to health resources. Younger and older individuals interested in issues of lifestyles, prevention, monitoring and wellbeing are now aware of available telemedicine and telehealth services.

At the individual level, internet-based information sources and services can provide individuals with insights regarding health concerns at any single point in time and over an extended period of time as well. In turn, users' involvement in social networks boosts their level of health literacy and leads them toward various health behaviors. Being aware of health-related products and services may alleviate the unpleasant symptoms of a health problem. Hence, online information offers the necessary resources to make people more willing to form new health habits and facilitates effective monitoring of patterns of change among individuals with health concerns. Moreover, eHealth information on the internet makes individuals more confident and increases their level of trust in human resources such as physicians, nurses and medical staff. Internet users seem to be more satisfied with contact with their physicians. Nonetheless, in order to maximize the benefits of online health information, users must first possess or acquire the necessary technological skills and develop the "right" frame of mind as manifested in their health attitudes. For these reasons, gaining an understanding of the challenges associated with the use of virtual source for health issues remains a significant endeavor.

One major and potential challenge posed by this process of health empowerment is the shift in the focus of medical care from "physician-centered" to "patient-centered". Physician-centered care advocates an authority based approach to healthcare whereas patient-centered care promotes an empowering approach. First, contrary to the authoritarian approach, today's health consumers ask physicians and nurses and other health professionals for advice and make use of support groups and online access to medical services. Second, health attitudes and personal health conditions play a central role in the extent to which individuals can and do make use of virtual sources of health. Third, situational effects in the individual's environment are highly likely to impede implementation of desired health regimes. Such conditions are often the outcome of contact with a particular health agent or health context. Specific health conditions such as a chronic illness motivate individuals to search online in order to retrieve relevant information. Access to relevant information increases understanding, making it easier to acquire a complete perspective on one's medical condition, treatment or medications, thereby increasing the chances of recovery. These situational factors underscore the importance of addressing both the benefits and the risks of using eHealth and mHealth sources of health information and disclose the sources of potential dysfunctions in the use of digital health. Consequently, the entire spectrum of individual-level characteristics associated with healthcare behaviors should be examined in the development of institutional healthcare and the initiation of healthcare reforms based on the increasing significance of virtual sources of health communication.

At the institutional level, illness prevention, early diagnosis and regular attention to a healthy lifestyle are significant factors in promoting public health. Health institutions and policymakers must encourage the development of services and programs that enable individuals to take more responsibility for their own health needs, diagnosis and treatment. The health sector is affected by the rapid development of information and communication technologies. Hence, online communication about health issues, including linking individuals in need of specific information and support with healthcare professionals, is becoming more common. In this sector, the information revolution has enabled health consumers and patients to access information on health and drugs. Nonetheless, several factors in the micro-macro association have become problematic.

First, the lack of direct contact when individuals seek health consultation through virtual devices significantly reduces the potential to treat patients holistically because such consultations are based on decisions that are "objective" for most people. As a result, despite the greater potential for quick and efficient outcomes, concerns also arise regarding the implications for professional responsibility and judgment, justice, autonomy, and trust. Second, the quality of virtual devices designed to address health concerns must be assessed, particularly since both individuals and institutional healthcare providers are using mobile applications more and more. Third, assessment of a health system must consider various public and private health agents as well as agents directly or indirectly involved with health behavior, such as health institutions, health insurance organizations and agents of health and safety legislation. Finally, inter-sectoral factors must be considered. For example, the Ministry of Education should promote education for women, and the Ministry of Welfare should encourage individuals to study new as well as traditional health professions.

Indeed, the macro-level policies of health systems and institutions should implement the principles of a satisficing solution in providing virtual services. These services should be effective in providing answers to disadvantaged individuals and social groups on the one hand and economically efficient on the other. Yet without overlooking issues of efficiency, health institutions must also address issues of effectiveness in order to increase the successful implementation of programs geared to illness prevention, early diagnosis and regular attention to a healthy lifestyle. Successfully combining all of these will prevent the generation and continuation of health divides while increasing health empowerment and successful self-management practices among those who need it most—the elderly, those situated in remote geographic areas and/or those facing chronic illness and disabilities. Being aware of the potential for "secondary level" digital divide effects and the ways to avoid them will increase the potential for health literacy and health empowerment.

Another issue gaining interest among all public and private institutional agents of health is how to combine between micro-level factors associated with the use of digital loci of health consumption and macro-level uses of these digital loci to provide health information and services. The wide range of these loci, which include health-related websites, participation in health forums, bulletin boards and health-related social networking sites, challenges the ability to provide a clear picture of the pros and cons of these sources for individual wellbeing. The difficult task of identifying successful associations between micro- and macro-level factors in digital health is affected by immediate changes.

On one hand, all these factors are interrelated, while on the other hand they are separated from each other in terms of institutional locus. As a result, while the role of health in establishing positive relationships is paramount in defining wellbeing, we still seek ways to increase wellness and quality of life, which are the classic antecedents of happiness. Nevertheless, individuals may not be aware of the significance of the micro-level behaviors that shape decision-making processes at the macro level. This is why we must reconsider and constantly evaluate ways to improve the collaborative and partnership relationships between patients, physicians and health systems in the context of the internet. Both the government and the health insurance companies should increase ICT use to provide reliable programs to all social groups as well as preventive and specialized information to minority groups. In addition, telemedicine (remote access to specialized physicians) should be considered as a means of diminishing ethnic inequalities in access to specialized care. The results can influence both policy and practice and, most importantly, benefit individual wellness and wellbeing.

Clearly, healthcare professionals should strive to ensure that their patients do not rely solely on digital media and should refer them to more credible sources. People with relevant expertise should teach individuals to combine information from different sources, such as healthcare professionals and/or members of service user organizations, so they can achieve effective self-management. Since technology is often regarded as a rational rather than an empathic means in many situations, human intervention should always be welcomed and encouraged. Human communication between healthcare professionals and their patients facilitates the expression of fears, concerns and difficult emotions by providing support and concrete steps to alleviate anxiety. Avoiding principles that consider health needs to be similar and not specific and understanding that skills are not universal constitute important steps in improving the relationship between the micro- and macro-level conditions for successful healthcare services. Doing so may be expensive in terms of emotional and physical resources on the part of institutional healthcare providers, but this remains the best way to ensure wise use of online and virtual sources of health information.

After all, both online and offline health management rely upon the assumption that individuals need and should seek a better quality of life. Some may see improved quality of life in terms of better life conditions, others may evaluate it in terms of better health and still others may define it as greater public accountability. Nevertheless, definitions of individual and institutional forms of health and wellbeing need to be aligned around notions of wellness and wellbeing, which in the past were related to happiness. While the role of health in establishing positive relationships is paramount in defining wellbeing, we still seek ways to increase wellness. Ultimately, the major research breakthrough can be seen in our renewed focus on quality of life and its classic antecedent—happiness.

CHAPTER 9

Conclusions

Today's information society is characterized by rapid information production, distribution, storage and access. Information and communication technologies facilitate easy and updated access to information for all individuals who have technological and computer skills and access to the internet. Everyday activities such as communicating with others, purchasing goods, banking, and searching for any kind of information are all available online. The health landscape has changed as well, such that in a growing number of societies access to medical information has changed dramatically and the pursuit of health today takes place within a widening network of online and offline sources.

Social media and social networks that address people's needs for health information and health services and support are part of eHealth and mHealth, which has emerged from growing use of the internet and social media. In case of a health problem, people use health professionals, family and the internet as important sources of information. Individuals now have a choice. They can consult a health professional, go online to pursue more information, and connect with online and offline social networks that include both health professionals and experienced patients. As the use of apps and technology-based tools for health concerns increases, so does the need to adopt an interdisciplinary approach to examine variations in the use of online health forums.

The purpose of this review is to discuss the factors associated with the use of online sources of health and the association between micro-level use of the internet for health purposes and macro-level challenges in promoting virtual sources of health products and health services. Individuals who have adopted the health empowerment approach take responsibility, ask questions and act upon the answers. Accessing health-related websites and participation in health forums, bulletin boards and health-related social networking sites now constitute a major path to health information and self-management of health concerns.

First, online searches enable individuals to search on their own time and at their own pace. Second, access to relevant information can shape individuals' understanding of their medical situation. Third, online health forums can increase the chances for recovery because they empower individuals to take the necessary steps to eliminate sources of concern. Indeed, understanding makes it easier todevelop a complete perspective on one's medical condition, treatment type or medications. Fourth, online health information provides the resources necessary to increase an individual's willingness to form new health habits. Finally, knowing about health-related products and services may alleviate the bothersome symptoms of a health problem and increase the use of available online health services. As a result, individuals are more likely to set health goals, make concrete plans and understand that some means are better facilitators than others in achieving a desired health target.

The empowered information control process can place the institutional healthcare provider in a role that is equal to that of the patients. Health consumers who come to their health provider armed with information they found on the web and preconceived notions about their diagnosis want to play an active role in therapeutic decisions even though they may be relying on misleading or misinterpreted health information. Seeking virtual sources of information may initially be related to individuals' lack of satisfaction and trust in institutional health strategies and lack of trust in the authoritarian health information control process.

Indeed, health attitudes and specific health conditions play a central role in the extent to which individuals can and do implement virtual sources of health information. Novel constructs such as privacy concerns, risk beliefs, self-efficacy and autonomy have taken their place alongside traditional psychology-related constructs such as extrinsic/intrinsic motivation and technology constructs such as ease of use and usefulness. Socioeconomic variations are important factors in determining technological skills and the extent of online health forum use. If these factors are disregarded, unsolicited use of online forums may increase the risk of generating and deepening differences in access and use of eHealth and mHealth services, especially among individuals facing difficult health challenges. Additional variations in technology use for health can be attributed to (a) types of health behaviors, which are still not thoroughly defined; (b) differences in motivations and circumstances underlying personal health decisions and behaviors; (c) the effects of ICT use on the patient-healthcare provider relationship; and (d) the effects of ICT-based communication on health attitudes and on ethical issues related to the adoption of virtual health services.

Due to these variations, the mere use of virtual sources and online forums such as online health services and social media cannot guarantee the adoption of healthy behaviors. Consequently, neither access nor use of the internet and other related online sources of health such as mobile health applications is similar for all individuals and all social groups. In fact, the rising number of online health information seekers in western societies has made it obvious that differences in access to online health information will affect individuals with lower technology skills. Indeed, individuals or groups who are disadvantaged in terms of their technology skills and/or access to online health information and services may disregard health issues, not ask for help and support, and have little motivation to deal with illness prevention. Hence, a lack of skills that leads to less use of online health information and services may result in poorer health practices. Thus, despite major investments in the development and introduction of advanced health services and programs, the effectiveness of these services is questionable because health literacy is still limited, in particular among the disadvantaged who need it most.

Health institutions need to address notions of effectiveness and efficiency in order to increase the successful implementation of programs for illness prevention, early diagnosis and regular attention to a healthy lifestyle, without disregarding the importance of individual-level factors. Adopting comprehensive health policy programs rather than focusing on on-the-spot technology-facilitated solutions to promote healthy lifestyles in disadvantaged communities has been shown to have a lower impact and outcome. This is due to environmental changes and a lack of consideration for anthropological variables (deSilva Sanigorski *et al.*, 2010). Without a multiple stakeholder approach, there is no basis for drawing conclusions about the effectiveness of the program or for deriving in-depth insights.

Recent studies promote adopting multilevel and multifaceted evaluation programs. Such programs should consider both the immediate short-range outcomes and the indirect long-range outcomes of health programs, especially when technology is involved. Moreover, such evaluations should be culturally diverse since these programs are often easily transferred from one nation to another and are thus subject to cultural factors. Programs and even policies often cannot be applied successfully to diverse settings and target groups. In fact, according to Broms (2019), the responsibility of social media for users' health may go beyond communications policies. Recent studies confirm that the public health risk posed by platforms such as Facebook goes deeper than content-level risks deriving from communications policies (Atroszko *et al.*, 2018; Guedes *et al.*, 2016). The for-profit orientation of these platforms means that the risk of user addiction is higher (Boweles, 2018). Hence, neither the quality nor the effective use of these online platforms is ideal in terms of several factors, among them health risks, ethical concerns and privacy (Lakshmanan, 2019). Stronger integration between healthcare providers in the public and private sectors is needed to ensure higher quality and less damage to health recipients. Public health researchers may not be satisfied with such a compromise.

An integrated healthcare system is apparently the best way to address the gaps between autonomous and unsolicited health information and to ensure a professional flow of information addressing patients' healthcare concerns. These solutions should be able to connect between the various healthcare agents and patients. They should include all relevant stakeholders, among them developers, data analysts, regulators and internet-based providers. On the whole, such an inclusive and interdisciplinary perspective will promote the introduction of and adherence to an ethical approach to the use of eHealth and mHealth devices and raise awareness of the impact of eHealth. Recent concerns reflect early developments in bioethics in the 1970s. The problems associated with the use of unsolicited and indirect contact with physicians have been the focus of a growing body of research that theoretically examines certain universal needs. Many technologies related to health are based on low accountability and a strong market orientation that strives to lower costs to institutional health systems.

The reasons underlying personal health decisions and behavior have not been properly evaluated. A great deal remains to be said and done in the area of person-to-person empathy. The potential appeasement and comfort provided by the authority of a specialist who understands that the body is a whole physical entity must be considered. Unaddressed symptoms that are often undetected by the patient himself may prove to be sources of discomfort or basic deficiencies in the individual's condition. Recent studies have in fact emphasized the importance of adopting comprehensive health policy programs rather than focusing on immediate solutions facilitated by technology.

References

Abel, T., Frohlich, K.L. (2012). Capitals and capabilities: linking structure and agency to reduce health inequalities. *Social Science & Medicine, 74*(2), 236-244.
[http://dx.doi.org/10.1016/j.socscimed.2011.10.028] [PMID: 22177750]

Abroms, L. C. (2019). Public health in the era of social media. *American Journal of Public Health, 109*(52), S130-S131.
[http://dx.doi.org/10.2105/AJPH.2018.304947]

Abroms, L. C., Gold, R. S., Allegrante, J. P. (2019). Promoting health on social media: The way forward. *Health Education and Behavior, 46*(2), 9-11.

Aceijas, C. (2011). *Assessing evidence to improve population health and wellbeing.* (pp. 3-16). UK: Exeter.

Ahadzadeh, A.S., Pahlevan Sharif, S., Ong, F.S., Khong, K.W. (2015). Integrating health belief model and technology acceptance model: an investigation of health-related internet use. *Journal of Medical Internet Research, 17*(2), e45.
[http://dx.doi.org/10.2196/jmir.3564] [PMID: 25700481]

Akbar, S., Coiera, E., Magrabi, F. (2020). Safety concerns with consumer-facing mobile health applications and their consequences: a scoping review. *Journal of the American Medical Informatics Association, 27*(2), 330-340.
[http://dx.doi.org/10.1093/jamia/ocz175] [PMID: 31599936]

Alas, A., Sajadi, K.P., Goldman, H.B., Anger, J.T. (2013). The rapidly increasing usefulness of social media in urogynecology. *Female Pelvic Medicine & Reconstructive Surgery, 19*(4), 210-213.
[http://dx.doi.org/10.1097/SPV.0b013e3182909872] [PMID: 23797519]

Albrecht, U-V. (2013). Transparency of health-apps for trust and decision making. *Journal of Medical Internet Research, 15*(12), e277.
[http://dx.doi.org/10.2196/jmir.2981] [PMID: 24449711]

Aljaber, T., Gordon, N. (2016). Evaluation of mobile health education applications for health pro- fessionals and patients. *Proceedings of the International Conference on E-Health, EH 2016 - Part of the Multi Conference on Computer Science and Information Systems 2016,* Funchal, Madeira107-114.

Alkhudairi, B., Pemberton, L. (2016). Factors affecting the acceptance of mHealth technology by Saudi diabetics and doctors. *Multi conference on computer science and information systems: eHealth,* Funchal, Madeira,199-202.

Allegrante, J.P., Elaine Auld, M. (2019). Advancing the Promise of Digital Technology and Social Media to Promote Population Health. *Health Education & Behavior, 46*(2S), 5S-8S.

Ancker, J.S., Barrón, Y., Rockoff, M.L., Hauser, D., Pichardo, M., Szerencsy, A., Calman, N. (2011). Use of an electronic patient portal among disadvantaged populations. *Journal of general internal medicine, 26*(10), 1117-1123.
[http://dx.doi.org/10.1007/s11606-011-1749-y] [PMID: 21647748]

Anderson, L., Ostrom, A.L. (2015). Transformative service research: Advancing our knowledge about service and well-being. *Journal of Service Research, 18*(3), 243-249.

[http://dx.doi.org/10.1177/1094670515591316]

Andoulsi, I., Wilson, P.P. (2013). Understanding liability in eHealth: towards greater clarity at European Union level. In: C, George, D, Whitehouse, P, Duquenoy, (Eds.), *eHealth: Legal, Ethical and Governance Challenges,* Heidelberg; New York: Springer.165-180.
[http://dx.doi.org/10.1007/978-3-642-22474-4_7]

Andreassen, H.K., Bujinowska, F., Chronaki, C.E., Dumitru, R.C., Pudule, I., Santana, S., Henning, V., Wynn, R. (2007). European Citizens' use of E-Health Services: A study of Seven Countries. *BMC Public Health.*

Andreotti, A., Anselmi, G., Eichhorn, T., Hoffmann, C.P., Micheli, M. (2017). European perspectives on participation in the sharing economy. *SSRN Electronic Journal.*
[http://dx.doi.org/10.2139/ssrn.3046550]

Antheunis, M.L., Tates, K., Nieboer, T.E. (2013). Patients' and health professionals' use of social media in health care: motives, barriers and expectations. *Patient Education and Counseling, 92*(3), 426-431.
[http://dx.doi.org/10.1016/j.pec.2013.06.020] [PMID: 23899831]

Aparicio-Martinez, P., Perea-Moreno, A.J., Martinez-Jimenez, M.P., Redel-Macías, M.D., Pagliari, C., Vaquero-Abellan, M. (2019). Social Media, Thin-Ideal, Body Dissatisfaction and Disordered Eating Attitudes: An Exploratory Analysis. *International Journal of Environmental Research and Public Health, 16*(21), 4177.
[http://dx.doi.org/10.3390/ijerph16214177] [PMID: 31671857]

Ariani, A., Koesoema, A.P., Soegijoko, S. (2017). Innovative healthcare applications of ict for developing countries. In: Qudrat-Ullah, H., Tsasis, P., (Eds.), *Innovative Healthcare Systems for the 21st Century. Understanding Complex Systems.* (pp. 15-70). Cham: Springer.
[http://dx.doi.org/10.1007/978-3-319-55774-8_2]

Arie, S (2015). Can mobile phones transform healthcare in low and middle income countries? *BMJ, 350,* h1975-h1975.
[http://dx.doi.org/10.1136/bmj.h1975]

Armstrong, N., Eborall, H. (2012). The sociology of medical screening: past, present and future. *Sociology of Health & Illness, 34*(2), 161-176.
[http://dx.doi.org/10.1111/j.1467-9566.2011.01441.x] [PMID: 22369578]

Ashill, N.J., Carruthers, J., Krisjanous, J. (2006). The effect of management commitment to service quality on frontline employees' affective and performance outcomes: An empirical investigation of the New Zealand public healthcare sector. *International Journal of Nonprofit Volunteer Sector Marketing, 11,* 271-287.
[http://dx.doi.org/10.1002/nvsm.281]

Atroszko, P.A., Balcerowska, J.M., Bereznowski, P., Biernatowska, A., Pallesen, S., Andreassen, C.S. (2018). Facebook addiction among polish undergraduate students: Validity of measurement and relationship with personality and well-being. *Computers in Human Behavior, 85,* 329-338.
[http://dx.doi.org/10.1016/j.chb.2018.04.001]

Bakker, D., Kazantzis, N., Rickwood, D., Rickard, N. (2016). Mental health smartphone apps: Review and evidence-based recommendations for uture developments. *JMIR Mental Health, 3*(1), e7.
[http://dx.doi.org/10.2196/mental.4984] [PMID: 26932350]

Bandura, A. (1997). *Self-Efficacy: The Exercise of control..* New York: Freeman.

Bandura, A. (2004). Health promotion by social cognitive means. *Health Education & Behavior, 31*(2), 143-

164.
[http://dx.doi.org/10.1177/1090198104263660] [PMID: 15090118]

Barak, A., Grohol, J.M. (2011). Current and future trends in Internet-supported mental health interventions. *Journal of Technology in Human Services, 29*(3), 155-196.
[http://dx.doi.org/10.1080/15228835.2011.616939]

Barak, A., Klein, B., Proudfoot, J.G. (2009). Defining Internet-supported therapeutic interventions. *Annals of Behavioral Medicine, 38*(1), 4-17.
[http://dx.doi.org/10.1007/s12160-009-9130-7]

Baran, S.J., Davis, D.K. (2000). Mass Communication Theory, Foundations, Ferment, and Future. CA: Wadsworth/Thomson Learning.

Barker, J.O., Rohde, J.A. (2019). Topic clustering of e-cigarette submissions among Reddit communities: A network perspective. *Health Education & Behavior, 46*(2_suppl), 59S-68S.
[http://dx.doi.org/10.1093/intqhc/13.4.317] [PMID: 11560351]

Baron-Epel, O., Dushenat, M., Friedman, N. (2001). Evaluation of the consumer model: relationship between patients' expectations, perceptions and satisfaction with care. *International Journal for Quality in Health Care, 13*(4), 317-323.

Batchelor, R., Bobrowicz, A., Mackenzie, R., Milne, A. (2012). Challenges of ethical and legal responsibilities when technologies' uses and users change: social networking sites, decision- making capacity and dementia. *Ethics and Information Technology, 14*(2), 99-108.
[http://dx.doi.org/10.1007/ s10676-012-9286-x]

Beckfield, J., Krieger, N. (2009). Epi+ demos+ cracy: linking political systems and priorities to the magnitude of health inequities—evidence, gaps, and a research agenda. *Epidemiologic reviews, 31*(1), 152-177.

Bekalu, M. A., McCloud, R. F., Viswanath, K. (2019). Association of social media use with social well-being, positive mental health, and self-rated health: disentangling routine use from emotional connection to use. *Health Education & Behavior, 46*(2_suppl), 69S-80S.

Bekalu, M. A., McCloud, R. F., Viswanath, K. (2019). Association of social media use with social well-being, positive mental health, and self-rated health: Disentangling routine use from emotional connection to use. *Health Education & Behavior, 46*(2_suppl), 69S-80S.

Benetoli, A., Chen, T.F., Aslani, P. (2018). How patients' use of social media impacts their interactions with healthcare professionals. *Patient Education and Counseling, 101*, 439-444.
[http://dx.doi.org/10.1016/j.pec.2017.08.015]

Bennett, L., Humphries, R. (2014). Making best use of the better care fund. *Spending to save?*. London: The King's Fund.

Bhambra, G.K., de Sousa Santos, B. (2017). Introduction: Global challenges for sociology. *Sociology, 51*, 3-10.
[http://dx.doi.org/10.1177/0038038516674665]

Bhattacherjee, A. (2001). Understanding information systems continuance: an expectation-confirmation model. *MIS quarterly, 25*, 351-370.

Biggs, J. (2016). Why bitcoin can't help the poorest—Yet. *Techcrunch.* https://techcrunch.com/2016 /01/10/why-bitcoin-cant-help-the-poorest-yet/

Black, K., Dobbs, D. (2013). Community-dwelling older adults' perceptions of dignity: core meanings, challenges, supports and opportunities. *Ageing and Society, 34*(8), 1292-1313.

Blank, G. (2013). Who creates content? *Information, Communication & Society, 16*(4), 590-612.

Blank, G., Groselj, D. (2014). The dimensions of Internet use: Amount, variety and types. *Information, Communication & Society, 17*(4), 417-435.

Blank, G., Lutz, C. (2017). Representativeness of social media in Great Britain: Investigating Facebook, Linkedin, Twitter, Pinterest, Google+, and Instagram. *American Behavioral Scientist, 61*(7), 741-756.

Blank, G., Lutz, C. (2018). Benefits and harms from Internet use: A differentiated analysis of Great Britain. *New Media & Society, 20*(2), 618-640.

Blank, R., Burau, V., Kuhlmann, E. (2017). Comparative health policy. *Macmillan International Higher Education.* London: Red Globe Press.

Blut, M., Wang, C., Schoefer, K. (2016). Factors influencing the acceptance of self-service technologies: A meta-analysis. *Journal of Service Research, 19*(4), 396-416.
[http://dx.doi.org/10.1177/1094670516662352]

Booker, C.L, Kelly, Y.J, Sacker, A (2018). Gender differences in the associations between age trends of social media interaction and well-being among 10-15 year olds in the UK. *BMC Public Health, 18*(1), 321.
[http://dx.doi.org/10.1186/s12889-018-5220-4]

Borzekowski, D. L. (2019). Constancy (the New Media "C") and future generations. *Health Education & Behavior, 46*(2_suppl), 20S-29S.

Bowles, C. (2018). *Ghosts of Willowbrook: Disability, Mourning, and Feminism (Doctoral dissertation, Central European University).*

Bradby, H. (2016). Research agenda in medical sociology. *Frontiers in Sociology, 1*, 14.
[http://dx.doi.org/10.3389/fsoc.2016.00014]

Bradby, H., Green, G., Davison, C., Krause, K. (2017). Is super diversity a useful concept in European medical sociology? *Frontiers in Sociology., 1*, 17.
[http://dx.doi.org/10.3389/fsoc.2016.00017]

Brake, D. (2014). Are we all online content creators now? Web 2.0 and digital divides. *Journal of Computer-Mediated Communication, 19*(3), 591-609.

Broom, A. (2005). Virtually healthy: The impact of Internet use on disease experience and the doctor-patient relationship. *Qualitative Health Research, 15*(3), 325-345.

Brusilovskiy, E., Townley, G., Snethen, G., Salzer, M.S. (2016). Social media use, community participation and psychological well-being among individuals with serious mental illnesses. *Computers in Human Behavior, 65*, 232-240.
[http://dx.doi.org/10.1016/j.chb.2016.08.036]

Bucher, T. (2017). The algorithmic imaginary: Exploring the ordinary affects of Facebook algorithms. *Information, Communication & Society, 20*(1), 30-44.

Büchi, M., Festic, N., Latzer, M. (2018). How social wellbeing is affected by digital inequalities. *International Journal of Communication, 12*, 3686-3706.

Bundorf, M.K., Wagner, T.H., Singer, S.J., Baker, L.C. (2006). Who searches the Internet for health information? *Health Services Research, 41*, 819-836.

Burau, V., Blank, R.H. (2006). Comparing health policy: an assessment of typologies of health systems. *Journal of comparative policy analysis, 8*(01), 63-76.

Burawoy, M. (2005). The return of the repressed: recovering the public face of U.S. sociology, one hundred years on. *The ANNALS of the American Academy of Political and Social Science, 600*, 68-85.
[http://dx.doi.org/10.1177/0002716205277028]

Busse, R. (2006). Gesundheitssysteme als epidemiologischer Gegenstand–oder: Wie wissen wir, wie effektiv Gesundheitssysteme sind? *Bundesgesundheitsblatt Gesundheitsforschung Gesundheitsschutz, 49*(7), 611-621.

Carrell, D., Ralston, J.D. (2006). Variation in adoption rates of a patient web portal with a shared medical record by age, gender, and morbidity level. *AMIA Annual Symposium Proceedings, 2006*, 871.

Casciaro, T., Piskorski, M.J. (2005). Power imbalance, mutual dependence and constraint absorption: Resource dependence theory revisited. *Administrative Science Quarterly, 50*(2), 167-199.

Casilari, E., Luque, R., Morón, M-J. (2015). Analysis of android device-based solutions for fall detection. *Sensors (Basel), 15*(8), 17827-17894.
[http://dx.doi.org/10.3390/s150817827]

Caspi, A., Chayut, E., Saporta, K. (2008). Participation in class and in online discussions: Gender differences. *Computers & Education, 50*(3), 718-724.10.1016/j.compedu.2006.08.003

Cavoukian, A., Castro, D. (2014). Big data and innovation, setting the record straight: de- identification does work. *Information and Privacy Commissioner.* Ontario, Canada. http://www2.itif.org/2014-big-data-deidentification.pdf

Chambers, R., Schmid, M., Birch-jones, J. (2016). *Digital healthcare: the essential guide..* Oxford: Otmoor Publishing.

Charani, E., Castro-Sánchez, E., Moore, L.S., Holmes, A. (2014). Do smartphone applications in health- care require a governance and legal framework? It depends on the application! *BMC Medicine, 12*(1), 29.
[http://dx.doi.org/10.1186/1741-7015-12-29]

Charters, E. (2003). The use of think-aloud methods in qualitative research—An introdction to think-aloud methods. *Brock Education, 12*(2), 68-82.
[http://dx.doi.org/10.26522/brocked.v12i2.38]

Chen, W., Lee, K.H. (2014). More than search? Informational and participatory eHealth behaviors. *Computers in Human Behavior, 30*, 103-109.
[http://dx.doi.org/10.1016/j.chb.2013.07.028]

Chen, W., Lee, K.H., Straubhaar, J.D., Spence, J. (2014). Getting a second opinion: Social capital, digital inequalities, and health information repertoires. *Journal of the Association for Information Science and Technology, 65*(12), 2552-2563.

Chew, F., Palmer, S., Kim, S. (1998). Testing the influence of the health belief model and a television program on nutrition behavior. *Health Communication, 10*(3), 227-245.
[http://dx.doi.org/10.1207/s15327027hc1003_3]

Chomutare, T., Fernandez-Luque, L., Årsand, E., Hartvigsen, G. (2011). Features of mobile diabetes applications: review of the literature and analysis of current applications compared against evidence-based guidelines. *Journal of Medical Internet Research, 13*(3), e65. [http://dx.doi.org/10.2196/jmir.1874]

Christakis, N.A., Fowler, J.H. (2013). Social contagion theory: examining dynamic social networks and human behavior. *Statistics in medicine, 32*(4), 556-577.

Christopherson, R. (2016). How do Alexa and Amazon Echo help disabled people? *Ability Net.* https://www.abilitynet.org.uk/news-blogs/how-do-alexa-and-amazon-echo-help-disabled-people

CIDA. (2000). CIDA Evaluation Guide.*Performance Review Branch.*

Clarke, M., Mars, M. (2015). An investigation into the use of 3G mobile communications to provide Telehealth Services in Rural KwaZulu-Natal. *Telemed E-Health, 21*(2), 115-119. [http://dx.doi.org/10.1089/tmj.2014.0079]

Clemensen, J., Danbjorg, D., Syse, M., Coxon, I. (2016). The rise of patient 3.0. The impact of social media. *8th International Conference on e-Health,* 1-3.

Conley, D., Springer, K.W. (2001). Welfare state and infant mortality. *Journal of Sociology, 107*(3), 768-807.

Correa, T. (2010). The participation divide among "online experts": Experience, skills and psychological factors as predictors of college students' web content creation. *Journal of Computer▯Mediated Communication, 16*(1), 71-92.

Cotten, S.R., Gupta, S.S. (2004). Characteristics of online and offline health information seekers and factors that discriminate between them. *Social Science and Medicine, 59*(9), 1795-1806. [http://dx.doi.org/10.1016/j.socscimed.2004.02.020]

Coughlin, S.S., Stewart, J.L., Young, L., Heboyan, V., De Leo, G. (2018). Health literacy and patient web portals. *International journal of medical informatics, 113*, 43-48.

Cristensen, C.M., Grossmans, J.H., Hwang, J.H. (2009). *The Innovator's prescription: a disruptive solu- tion for health care..* New York: McGraw-Hill Education.

Cund, A, Connolly, P, Birch-Jones, J, Kay, M (2015). *The Innovator's prescription: a disruptive solution for health care.* New York: McGraw-Hill Education.

Currie, S.L., Mcgrath, P.J., Day, V. (2010). Development and usability of an online CBT program for symptoms of moderate depression, anxiety, and stress in post-secondary students. *Computers in Human Behavior, 26*(6), 1419-1426. [http://dx.doi.org/10.1016/j.chb.2010.04.020]

Dai, S.M. (2020). An adaptive computation offloading mechanism for mobile health applications. *IEEE Transactions on Vehicular Technology, 69*(1), 998-1007.

Darkins, A.W., Cary, M.A. (2000). Telemedicine and telehealth: principles, policies, performances and pitfalls. Berlin, Heidelberg: Springer.

Daskin, M.S., Dean, L.K., Sainfort&, F., P.Pierskalla, W. (2004). Location of health care facilities in Braudeau. *Operation Research and Healthcare, 46-82.*

Davis, F.D. (1989). Perceived usefulness, perceived ease of use, and user acceptance of information technology. *MIS quarterly,* 319-340.

Davis, S.E., Osborn, C.Y., Kripalani, S., Goggins, K.M., Jackson, G.P. (2015). Health literacy, education levels, and patient portal usage during hospitalizations. *AMIA Annual Symposium Proceedings, 2015,* 1871.

de los Reyes, G., Jr (2019). Institutional entrepreneurship for digital public health promotion: Challenges and opportunities. *Health Education & Behavior, 46*(2_suppl), 30S-36S.

de Silva-Sanigorski, AM., Bolton, K., Haby, M., Kremer, P., Gibbs, L. (2010). Scaling up community-based obesity prevention in Australia: background and evaluation design of the Health Promoting Communities: Being Active Eating Well initiative. *BMC public health, 10,* 65.

Degli Esposti, S. (2014). When big data meets dataveillance: the hidden side of analytics. *Surveillance & Society, 12*(2), 209-225. http://library.queensu.ca/ojs/index.php/surveillance-and-society/article/view/analytics/analytic

Delbanco, S. (2009). Using technology to improve quality and patient safety. *Healthcare Financial Management,* (December), 42-45.

Deng, L., Turner, D.E., Gehling, R., Prince, B. (2010). User experience, satisfaction, and continual usage intention of IT. *European Journal of Information Systems, 19*(1), 60-75.

Department of Health. (2013). The mandate. *A mandate from the Government to the NHS Commissioning Board.* London.

Dholakia, U.M., Bagozzi, R.P., Pearo, L.K. (2004). A social influence model of consumer participation in network- and small-group-based virtual communities. *International Journal of Research in Marketing, 21*(3), 241-263.
[http://dx.doi.org/10.1016/j.ijresmar.2003.12.004]

Diaz, J.A., Griffith, R.A., Ng, J.J., Reinert, S.E., Friedmann, P.D., Moulton, A.W. (2002). Patients' use of the Internet for medical information. *Journal of General Internal Medicine, 17*(3), 180-185.

DiMaggio, P., Bonikowski, B. (2008). Make money surfing the web? The impact of Internet use on the earnings of U.S. workers. *American Sociological Review, 73,* 227-250.

DiMaggio, P., Hargittai, E., Celeste, C., Shafer, S. (2004). Digital inequality: From unequal access to differentiated use. In: Neckerman, K., (Ed.), *Social Inequality* (pp. 355-400). New York, NY: Russell Sage Foundation.

Dobransky, K., Hargittai, E. (2012). Inquiring minds acquiring wellness: Uses of online and offline sources for health information. *Health Communication, 27*(4), 331-343.
[http://dx.doi.org/10.1080/10410236.2011.585451]

Dodel, M., Mesch, G. (2018). Inequality in digital skills and the adoption of online safety behaviors. *Information, Communication & Society, 21*(5), 712-728.
[http://dx.doi.org/10.1080/1369118X.2018.1428652]

Döhler, M., Manow, P. (1995). Kapitel 5 Staatliche Reformpolitik und die Rolle der Verbände im Gesundheitssektor. *Gesellschaftliche Selbstregelung und politische Steuerung, 23,* 140.

Donaldson, S.I., Gooler, L.E., Scriven, M. (2002). Strategies for managing evaluation anxiety: Toward a psychology of program evaluation. *American Journal of Evaluation, 23*(3), 261-272.

Dowling, M., Rickwood, D. (2016). Exploring hope and expectations in the youth mental health online counselling environment. *Computers in Human Behavior, 55*, 62-68. [http://dx.doi.org/10.1016/j.chb.2015.08.009]

Dubois, E., Ford, H. (2015). Qualitative political communication| trace interviews: An actorcentered approach. *International Journal of Communication, 9*, 2067-2091.

Duffy, B.E., Pruchniewska, U., Scolere, L. (2017). Platformspecific selfbranding: Imagined affordances of the social media ecology. *Proceedings of the 8th International Conference on Social Media & Society,* New York, NYACM.1-9.

Dutta, M.J., Bodie, G.D. (2008). Web searching for health: Theoretical foundations and connections to health related outcomes. In: Spink, A., Zimmer, M., (Eds.), *Web searching: Interdisciplinary perspectives.* New York: Peter Lang Publishing.

Dutta-Bergman, M. (2004). Developing a profile of consumer intention, to seek out health information beyond the doctor. *Health Marketing Quarterly, 21*, 91-112. a

Dutta-Bergman, M. (2004). Primary sources of health information: comparison in the domain of health attitudes, health cognition and health behaviors. *Health Communication, 16*, 273-288. b

Dutta-Bergman, M. (2004). The impact of completeness and web use motivation on the credibility of health information. *Journal of Communication, 54*, 253-269. c

Dutta-Bergman, M. (2004). Health attitudes, health cognitions among Internet health information seekers: Population based survey. *Journal of Medical Internet Research, 6*, 15. http://www.jmir.org/2004/2e15/index.htm

Dutta-Bergman, M. (2006). Media use theory and internet use for health care. In: Murero, M, Rice, E., (Eds.), *The Internet and Health Care: Theory, Research and Practice.* (pp. 83-103). Mahwah, NJ: Lawrence Erlbaum Associates.

Eikemo, T.A., Bambra, C., Judge, K., Ringdal, K. (2008). Welfare state regimes and differences in self-perceived health in Europe: a multilevel analysis. *Social science & medicine, 66*(11), 2281-2295.

Eisenberg, M., Berkowtz, (2009). *The big approach to information literacy skills.* http://www.bigsix.com

Emmanouilidou, M. (2016). The status of mHealth in Europe and a review of regulative challenges. *Multi conference on computer science and information systems: eHealth* (pp. 203-206). Funchal, Madeira.

des Borde, J.K.A., Foreman, J., Westrich-Robertson, T., Lopez-Olivo, M.A., Peterson, S.K., Hofstetter, C., Lyddiatt, A., Willcockson, I., Leong, A., Suarez-Almazor, M.E. (2020). Interactions and perceptions of patients with rheumatoid arthritis participating in an online support group. *Clinical rheumatology, 39*(6), 1775-1782.

Eslami, M., Rickman, A., Vaccaro, K., Aleyasen, A., Vuong, A., Karahalios, K. (2015). I always assumed that I wasn't really that close to [her]: Reasoning about invisible algorithms in news feeds. *CHI'15: Proceedings of the 33rd annual ACM conference on human factors in computing systems,* New York, NYACM.153-162.

Eugenio Mantovani and Pedro Cristobal Bocos E. Mantovani. (2017). *Are mHealth Apps Safe? The Intended Purpose Rule, Its Shortcomings and the Regulatory Options Under the EU Medical Device Framework.*Belgium: Springer.

[http://dx.doi.org/10.1007/978-3-319-60672-9_12]

European Commission. (2014). *Green paper on mobile health.* http://ec.europa.eu/newsroom /dae/document.cfm?doc_id=5147

European Commission. (2014). *EU consultation on mHealth.* https://ec.europa.eu/digital -single-market/en/public-consultation-green-paper-mobile-health

European Commission. (2016). *Market surveillance and vigilance.* https://eu/growth/sectors/medical-devices/market-surveil lance_en

European Commission. (2016). *MEDDEV 2.1/6 guidelines on the qualification and classification of stand alone software used in healthcare within the regulatory framework of medical devices.* http://www.twobirds.com/~/media/pdfs/news/articles/2016/firstdraftguidelinesandannexes.pdf?la=en

European Commission. (2016). *EU guidelines on assessment of the reliability of mobile health applications.EU guidelines on assessment of the reliability of mobile health applications.* http://ec.europa.eu/newsroom/dae/document.cfm?action=display&doc_id=16090

European Commission. (2016). *Code of conduct on privacy in mHealth.* http://ec.europa.eu/news-room/dae/document.cfm?action=display&doc_id=16125

European Commission. (2014). *Commission staff working document on the existing EU legal framework applicable to lifestyle and wellbeing apps.* Brussels.

European Commission. (2012). *eHealth Action Plan 2012–2020 – Innovative healthcare for the 21st century (2012), Brussels.*

European Union. (2016). *Treaty on the functioning of the European union.* http://eur-lex.europa.

Evans, W. D., Thomas, C. N., Favatas, D., Smyser, J., Briggs, J. (2019). Digital segmentation of priority populations in public health. *Health Education & Behavior, 46*(2_suppl), 81S-89S.

Eysenbach, G. (2009). Medicine 2.0: Social networking, collaboration, participation, apomediation, and openness. *Medical Internet Research, 10*(3), e22.

Ezendam, N. P., Noordegraaf, A., Kroeze, W., Brug, J., Oenema, A. (2013). Process evaluation of a computer-tailored intervention to prevent excessive weight gain among Dutch adolescents. *Health Promotion International, 28*(1), 26-35.

Ferguson, T. (2000). Online patient-helpers and physicians working together: a new partnership for high quality health care. *BMJ, 321*, 1129-1132.

Ferguson, T. (2008). E-patients: how they can help us heal healthcare. In: Earp, J.A., French, E.A., Gilkey, M.B., (Eds.), *Patient advocacy for health care quality: Strategies for achieving patient-centered care* (pp. 93-121). Massachusetts: Jones and Bartlett Publishers.

Figueras, J., Saltman, R. B., Busse, R., Dubois, H. F. (2004). Patterns and performance in social health insurance systems. *Series editors' introduction, 81*

Firth, J., Torous, J., Nicholas, J., Carney, R., Rosenbaum, S., Sarris, J. (2017). Can smartphone mental health interventions reduce symptoms of anxiety? A meta analysis of randomized controlled trials. *Journal of Affective Disorders, 218*, 15-22.https://doi-org.ezproxy.haifa.ac.il/10.1016/j.jad.2017.04.046

Forsström, J. (1997). Why certification of medical software would be useful? *International Journal of*

Medical Informatics, 47(3), 143-151.

Fox, N.J., Ward, K.J., O'Rourke, A.J. (2005). The expert patient: empowerment of medical dominance? The case of weight loss, pharmaceutical drugs and the internet. *Social Science & Medicine, 60*(6), 1299-1309.

Fox, S., Jones, S. (2009). The social life of health information. *Pew and American Life Project.* http://www.pewinternet.org/Reports/2009/8-The-Social-Life-of-Health-Information.aspx

Fox, S., Fallows, D. (2003). Internet health resources. *Pew Internet and American Life Project.*http://www.pewinternet.org.

Fox, S., Rainie, L. (2002). The online health care revolution. *Pew internet and American life project.*

Fraccaro, V., Balatsoukas, B., Peek, V. D. V. (2017). Patient portal adoption rates: a systematic literature review and meta-analysis. *Studies in health technology and informatics, 245*, 79-83.

Freeman, R. (2000). *The politics of health in Europe.* UK: Manchester University Press.

Fuchal, Madeira (2010). Same game, different rules? Gender differences in political participation. *Sex Roles, 62*(5-6), 318-333.
[http://dx.doi.org/10.1007/s11199-009-9729-y]

Gauld, R. (2009). *The new health policy..* UK: McGraw-Hill Education.

Gelissen, J. (2002). *Worlds of welfare, worlds of consent? Public opinion on the welfare state.* Netherlands: Brill.

George, C., Whitehouse, D., Duquenoy, P. (2013). *Assessing legal, ethical and governance challenges in eHealth* (pp. 3-22). Berlin, Heidelberg: Springer. http://link.springer.com/10.1007/978-3-642-22474-4

Ghobakhloo, M., Zulkifli, N.B., Aziz, F.A. (2010). The interactive model of user information technology acceptance and satisfaction in small and medium-sized enterprises. *European. European Journal of economics, finance and administrative sciences, 19*(1), 7-27.

Giaimo, S., Manow, P. (1999). Adapting the welfare state: the case of health care reform in Britain, Germany, and the United States. *Comparative Political Studies, 32*(8), 967-1000.

Gibbons, M.C. (2008). eHealth: Solutions for healthcare disparities. *Science + Business Media, LLC.* Berlin: Springer.

Gill, P., Kamath, A., Gill, T.S. (2012). Distraction: an assessment of smartphone usage in health care work settings. *Risk Manag Healthcare Policy, 105*
[http://dx.doi.org/10.2147/RMHP.S34813]

Gimenez-Perez, G., Gallach, M., Acera, E., Prieto, A., Carro, O., Orrega, E., Conzalez-Clemente, J.M., Mauricio, D. (2002). Evaluation of accessibility and use of new communication technologies in patients with type 1 diabetes mellitus. *Journal of Medical Internet Research, 4*(3), e16.

Ginossar, T., Nelson, S. (2010). La Comunidad Habla: using internet community-based information interventions to increase empowerment and access to health care of low income Latino immigrants. *Communication Education, 59.3*, 328-3244.

Gitau, S., Marsden, G., Donner, J. (2010). After access: Challenges facing mobileonly Internet users in the developing world. *Proceedings of the SIGCHI conference on human factors in computing systems,* New York, NYACM.2603-2606.

Giunti, G., Baum, A., Giunta, D., Plazzotta, F., Benitez, S., Gómez, A., González Bernaldo de Quiros, F. (2015). Serious games: a concise overview on what they are and their potential applications to healthcare. In: Sarkar, IN, Georgiou, A., Mazzoncini de Azevedo Marques, P., (Eds.), *eHealth-enabled health: proceedings of the 15ᵗʰ world congress on health and biomedical informatics* (pp. 386-390). Sao Paulo: IOS Press.

Giveon, S., Yaphe, J., Hekselman, I., Mahamid, S., Hermoni, D. (2009). Survey of doctors' experience of patients using the internet. *The Israel Medical Association Journal, 11*, 537-541.

Goldman, D., Smith, J.P. (2011). The increasing value of education to health. *Social Science & Medicine, 72*(10), 1728-1737.

Golle, P. (2006). Revisiting the uniqueness of simple demographics in the US population. *Proceedings of the 5th ACM workshop on Privacy in electronic society (WPES '06).,* York, NY, USA: Association for Computing Machinery.77-80.
[http://dx.doi.org/10.1145/1179601.1179615]

Goodman, M. (2016). *Future crimes: inside the digital underground and the battle for our connected world.* Toronto: Anchor Books.

Goodyear-Smith, F., Buetow, S. (2001). Power issues in the doctor-patient relationship. *Health Care Analysis, 9*, 449-462.

Play, Google (2013). *COPD – NHS decision aid.* https://play.google.com/store/apps/details?id=uk. co.activata.TotallyHealth.condition119

Play, Google (2016). *Telemed.* https://play.google.com/store/apps/details?id=com.telemed.ae&hl=es

Government Office for Science. (2014). The internet of things: making the most of the second digital revolution. *A report by the UK Government Chief Scientific Adviser.* London.

Graafland, M., Dankbaar, M., Mert, A., Lagro, J., De Wit-Zuurendonk, L., Schuit, S. (2014). How to systematically assess serious games applied to health care. *JMIR Serious Games, 2*(2), e11.
[http://dx.doi.org/10.2196/games.3825]

Grau, S., Kleiser, S., Bright, L. (2019). Exploring social media addiction among student Millennials. *Qualitative Market Research: An International Journal, 22*(2), 200-216.

Gray, K., Gilbert, C. (2018). Digital health research methods and tools: suggestions and selected resources for researchers. In: Holmes, D., Jain, L., (Eds.), *Advances in Biomedical Informatics. Intelligent Systems Reference Library* (Vol. 137). Cham: Springer.

Greenough, J. (2015). *How the "Internet of Things" will impact consumers, businesses, and governments in 2016 and beyond.* http://www.techinsider.io/

Grönroos, C. (2006). Adopting a service logic for marketing. *Marketing Theory, 6*(3), 317-333.
[http://dx.doi.org/10.1177/1470593106066794]

Guedes, E., Sancassiani, F., Carta, M.G., Campos, C., Machado, S., King, A.L.S., Nardi, A.E. (2016). Internet addiction and excessive social networks use: what about Facebook? *Clinical Practice and Epidemiology in Mental Health: CP & EMH, 12*, 43.

Gui, M., Argentin, G. (2011). Digital skills of Internet natives: Different forms of digital literacy in a random sample of northern Italian high school students. *New Media & Society, 13*(6), 963-980.

Gümüş, R., Sönmez, Y. (2020). Quality of online communication tools at hospitals and their effects on health service consumers' preferences. *International Journal of Healthcare Management,* *13*(1), 35-44.

Gurak, L.J., Hudson, B.L. (2006). E-Health: Trends and Theory. In: Rice, R., Murero, M., (Eds.), *The Internet and Health Care: Theory, Research and Practice.* UK: Routledge.

Hacker, J.S. (1998). The historical logic of national health insurance: structure and sequence in the development of British, Canadian, and US medical policy. *Studies in American Political Development, 12*(1), 57-130.

Hadwich, K., Georgi, G., Tuzovi, S., Buttner, J., Bruhn, M. (2009). Perceived quality of e-health services: A conceptual and empirical study of e-health services quality based on the C-OAR-SE Approach,in Straus. In: Brown, B.S., Edwardson, B., Johnston, R., (Eds.), *QUIS 11: Moving forward with service quality,* 183-186.

Halford, S., Savage, M. (2010). Reconceptualizing digital social inequality. *Information, Communication & Society, 13*(7), 937-955.

Hanlon, B, Thiel, S (2016). *The mobile health application revolution: tapping its potential.* http://www.covance.com/content/dam/covance/assetLibrary/whitepapers/Mobile-Health-Applications-WPC VD002-0816.pdf

Hardt, J.H., Hollis-Sawyer, L. (2007). Older adults seeking healthcare information on the Internet. *Educational Gerontology, 33,* 561-572.

Hargitai, E., Hsie, P.L. (2010). Predictors and consequences of differentiated practices on social network sites. *Information, Communication and Society, 13*(4), 515-536.

Hargittai, E., Hinnant, A. (2008). Digital inequality differences in young adults 'use of the Internet. *Communication Research, 35*(1), 602-621.

Hargittai, E. (2007). Whose space? Differences among users and nonusers of social network sites. *Journal of Computer-Mediated Communication, 13*(1), 276-297.

Hargittai, E. (2010). Digital na(t)ives? Variation in Internet skills and uses among members of the "net generation". *Sociological Inquiry, 80*(1), 92-113.

Hargittai, E. (2015). Is bigger always better? Potential biases of big data derived from social network sites. *The Annals of the American Academy of Political and Social Science, 659*(1), 63-76.

Hargittai, E., Hinnant, A. (2008). Digital inequality: Differences in young adults' use of the Internet. *Communication Research, 35*(5), 602-621.

Hargittai, E., Walejko, G. (2008). The participation divide: Content creation and sharing in the digital age. *Information, Communication & Society, 11*(2), 239-256.

Hartmann, C. W., Sciamanna, C. N., Blanch, D. C., Mui, S., Lawless, H., Manocchia, M., Rosen, R.K., Pietropaoli, A. (2007). A website to improve asthma care by suggesting patient questions for physicians: qualitative analysis of user experiences. *Journal of Medical Internet Research, 9*(1), e3.

Hassenteufel, P., Smyrl, M., Genieys, W., Moreno-Fuentes, F.J. (2010). Programmatic actors and the transformation of European health care states. *Journal of Health Politics, Policy and Law, 35*(4), 517-538.

Haug, M.R., Lavin, B. (1981). Practitioner or patient – Who is in charge? *Journal of Health and Social Behavior, 22,* 212-229.

Hawley, A.H. (1986). *Human ecology: a theoretical essay.*. Chicago: University of Chicago Press.

Heath, M., Porter, T.H. (2017). Patient health records: An exploratory study of patient satisfaction. *Health Policy Technol., 6*(4), 401-409.

Stallman, H.M. (2019). Efficacy of the my coping plan mobile application in reducing distress: A randomised controlled trial. *Clinical Psychologist., 23*(3), 206-212.

Hendrie, G.A., Hussain, M.S., Brindal, E., James-Martin, G., Williams, G., Crook, A. (2020). Impact of a mobile phone app to increase vegetable consumption and variety in adults: large-scale community cohort study. *JMIR Mhealth Uhealth, 8*(4), e14726.

Higgs, P., Gilleard, C. (2015). Rethinking old age. *Theorising the Fourth Age.* London: Palgrave Macmillan.

Hildebrandt, M. (2015). *Smart technologies and the end(s) of law: novel entanglements of law and technology.* Cheltenham: Edward Elgar Publishing.

Hilts, A., Parsons, C., Knockel, J. (2016). Every step you fake: a comparative analysis of fitness tracker privacy and security. *Open Effect Report.*https://openeffect.ca/reports/Every_Step_You_Fake.pdf

Hoffmann, C.P., Lutz, C., Meckel, M. (2015). Content creation on the Internet: A social cognitive perspective on the participation divide. *Information, Communication & Society, 18*(6), 696-716.

Holmes, M., Bishop, F.L., Calman, L. (2017). "I just googled and read everything": Exploring breast cancer survivors' use of the internet to find information on complementary medicine. *Complementary Therapies in Medicine, 33*, 78-84.

Househ, M., Borycki, E., Kushniruk, A. (2014). Empowering patients through social media: The benefits and challenges. *Health Informatics Journal, 20*(1), 50-58. http://www.openmhealth.org [http://dx.doi.org/10.1177/1460458213476969]

Huckvale, P, Tilney, B (2015). Unaddressed privacy risks in accredited health and wellness apps: a cross-sectional systematic assessment. *BMC Medicine, 13*, 214.

Huerta, TR, Walker, DM, Ford, EW (2016). An evaluation and ranking of children's hospital websites in the USA. *Journal of Medical Internet Research, 18*(8), e228.

Humphreys, L., Von Pape, T., Karnowski, V. (2013). Evolving mobile media: Uses and conceptualizations of the mobile Internet. *Journal of Computer☐Mediated Communication, 18*(4), 491-507.

Husereau, D., Drummond, M., Petrou, S. (2013). Consolidated health economic evaluation reporting standards statement. *Journal of Medical Economics, 16*(6), 713-719. [http://dx.doi.org/10.3111/13696998.2013.784591]

Igarashi, T., Takai, J., Yoshida, T. (2005). Gender differences in social network development *via* mobile phone text messages: A longitudinal study. *Journal of Social and Personal Relationships, 22*(5), 691-713. [http://dx.doi.org/10.1177/0265407505056492]

Ignatow, G., Robinson, L. (2017). Pierre Bourdieu: Theorizing the digital. *Information, Communication & Society, 20*(7), 950-966.

IHS report. (2013). *The world market for sports & fitness monitors.*

Immergut, E.M. (1992). *Health politics: interests and institutions in Western Europe.* UK: Cambridge

University Press.

International Telecommunications Union. (2014). *Filling the gap: legal and regulatory challenges of mobile health (mHealth) in Europe.* https://www.itu.int/en/ITU-D/Regional-Presence/Europe/Documents/ITU%20mHealth%20Regulatory%20gaps%20Discussion%20Paper%20June2014.pdf

International Telecommunications Union. (2017). *ICT facts and figures.* Geneva. https://www.itu.int/en/ITU-D/Statistics/Documents/facts/ICTFactsFigures2017.pdf

Irizarry, T., Dabbs, A.D., Curran, C.R. (2015). Patient portals and patient engagement: a state of the science review. *Journal of Medical Internet Research, 17*(6), e148.

Islam, Muhammad Nazrul, Karim, Md. Mahboob, Inan, Toki Tahmid, Islam, A. K. M. Najmul (2020). Investigating usability of mobile health applications in Bangladesh. *BMC Medical Informatics and Decision Making, 20*, 19.

ITU. (2015). *m-Powering development initiative: a report by the m-Powering development ini- tiative advisory board.* http://www.itu.int/en/ITU-D/Initiatives/m-Powering/Documents/m-PoweringDevelopment Initiative_Report2015.pdf

Itunes. (2015). *Self-help for anxiety management.* https://itunes.apple.com/us/app/self-help-for- anxiety-management/id666767947?mt=8

Iverson, S.A., Howard, K.B., Penney, B.K. (2008). Impact of Internet use on health related behaviors and the patient physician relationship: A survey-based study and review. *Journal of the American Osteopath Association, 108*, 699-711.

Jacobs, L., Marmor, T., Oberlander, J. (1999). The Oregon Health Plan and the political paradox of rationing: what advocates and critics have claimed and what Oregon did. *Journal of Health Politics, Policy and Law, 24*(1), 161-180.

Jaeger, M.M. (2016). Are the 'deserving needy' really deserving everywhere? cross-cultural heterogeneity and popular support for the old and the sick in eight western countries. *Social Justice, Legitimacy and the Welfare State.* (pp. 91-112). UK: Routledge.

Johnson, A. C., Lipkus, I., Tercyak, K. P., Luta, G., Rehberg, K., Phan, L., Mays, D. (2019). Development and pretesting of risk-based mobile multimedia message content for young adult hookah use. *Health Education & Behavior, 46*(2_suppl), 97S-105S.

Johnson, K.F., Kalkbrenner, M.T. (2017). The utilization of technological innovations to support college student mental health: Mobile health communication. *Journal of Technology in Human Services, 35*(4), 314-339.
[http://dx.doi.org/10.1080/15228835.2017.1368428]

Jönsson, B., Musgrove, P. (1997). Government financing. *Proceedings of a World Bank Conference,* World Bank Publications. *365*, 41.

Joseffson, U. (2006). Patient's online information-seeking behavior. In: Rice, R., Murero, M., (Eds.), *The Internet and Health Care: Theory, Research and Methods.* (pp. 127-149). UK: Routledge.

Kakai, H., Maskarinec, G., Shumay, D.M., Tatsumura, Y., Tasaki, K. (2003). Ethnic differences in choices of health information by cancer patients using complementary and alternative medicine: An exploratory study with correspondence analysis. *Social Science & Medicine, 56*(4), 851-862.

Kaler, L.S., Stebleton, M.J., Potts, C. (2020). It makes me feel even worse: empowering first-year women to

reconsider social media's impact on mental health. *About Campus, 24*(6), 10-17.
[http://dx.doi.org/10.1177/1086482219899650]

Kamerow, D (2013). Regulating medical apps: which ones and how much? *BMJ, 347*, f6009-f6009.

Kanavos, P., McKee, M. (1998). Macroeconomic constraints and health challenges facing health systems in the European Region. *Critical Challenges for Healthcare Reform, 23*-52.

Kapilashrami, A., Hill, S., Meer, N. (2015). What can health inequalities researchers learn from an intersectionality perspective? Understanding social dynamics with an inter-categorical approach. *Social Theory & Health, 13*, 288-307.
[http://dx.doi.org/10.1057/sth.2015.16]

Karvonen, S., Kestilä, L.M., Mäki-Opas, T.E. (2018). Who needs the sociology of health and illness? a new agenda for responsive and interdisciplinary sociology of health and medicine. *Frontiers in Sociology, 3*, 4.
[http://dx.doi.org/10.3389/fsoc.2018.00004]

Katz, J., Aspden, P. (2001). Networked communication practices and the security and privacy of electronic health care records. In: Rice, R., Katz, J., (Eds.), *The internet and health communication* (pp. 417-430). Thousand Oaks, CA: Sage.

Katz, J.R.R., Acord, S. (2004). E-health networks and social transformations: Expectations of centralization, experiences of decentralization. In: Castells, M., (Ed.), *The Network Society: A cross-cultural perspective* (pp. 298-319). Cheltenham, UK: Edward Elgar Publishing.

Kearney, M. D., Selvan, P., Hauer, M. K., Leader, A. E., Massey, P. M. (2019). Characterizing HPV vaccine sentiments and content on Instagram. *Health Education & Behavior, 46*(2_suppl), 37S-48S.

Kelson, J.N., Lam, M.K., Keep, M., Campbell, A.J. (2017). Development and evaluation of an online acceptance and commitment therapy program for anxiety: Phase I iterative design. *Journal of Technology in Human Services, 35*(2), 135-151.
[http://dx.doi.org/10.1080/15228835.2017.1309311]

Kendall Roundtree, A. (2017). Social health content and activity on Facebook: A survey study. *Journal of Technical Writing and Communication, 47*(3), 300-329.
[http://dx.doi.org/10.1177/0047281616641925]

Keogh, B (2012). *Poly implant Protheses(PIP) breast implants: interim report of the expert group.* http://www.nhs.uk/news/2012/01January/Documents/pip-report.pdfhttp://www.knmg.

Khuderia, S. (2016). *Intechnic, 12 Best Hospital and healthcare Websites.* https://www.intechnic. com/blog/12-best-hospital-and-healthcare-websites/

Kim, H., Zhang, Y. (2015). Health information seeking of low socioeconomic status Hispanic adults using smartphones. *Aslib Journal of Information Management, 67*(5), 542-561.

Kirch, W. (2008). Health belief model. *Encyclopedia of Public Health.* Netherlands: Springer.

Klein, R. (1997). Learning from others: shall the last be the first? *Journal of Health Politics, Policy and Law, 22*(5), 1267-1278.

Korp, P. (2006). Health on the internet: implications for health promotion. *Health Education Research, 21*(1), 78-86.

Korup, S., Szydlik, M. (2005). Causes and trends of the digital divide. *European Sociological Review, 21*(4),

409-422.

Kozica, S.L., Lombard, C.B., Hider, K., Harrison, C.L., Teede, H.J. (2015). Developing comprehensive health promotion evaluations: a methodological review. *MOJ Public Health,* 2(1), 00007. [http://dx.doi.org/10.15406/mojph.2015.02.00007]

Kramer, D.B., Xu, S., Kesselheim, A.S. (2012). Regulation of medical devices in the United States and European Union. *New England journal of medicine,* 366(9), 848-855.

Kushniruk, A. (2002). Evaluation in the design of health information systems: Application of approaches emerging from usability engineering. *Computers in Biology and Medicine,* 32(3), 141-149. [http://dx.doi.org/10.1016/s0010-4825(02)00011-2]

Kutzin, J. (2010). Conceptual framework for analysing health financing systems and the effects of reforms. *Implementing Health Financing Reform.*World Health Organization.

Kutzin, J., Cashin, C., Jakab, M., Fidler, A., Menabde, N. (2010). Implementing health financing reform in CE/EECCA countries: synthesis and lessons earned. *Implementing Health Financing Reform,* 383.

Kvasny, L. (2006). Cultural (re)production of digital inequality in a US community technology initiative. *Information, Communication & Society,* 9(2), 160-181.

Lafontaine, C. (2016). My body, my capital. Bio-citizenship in the era of Neoliberalism. *Plenary at the 16th European Society for Health and Medical Sociology Conference.*Geneva

Lakshmanan, R. YouTube is making it easier to remove recommendations you don't like. (2019). https://thenextweb.com/google/2019/06/27/youtube-is-making-it-easier-to-remove-recommen-ations-you-dont-like.

Lambert, S., Loiselle, C.G. (2007). Health information seeking behavior. *Qualitative Health Research,* 17(8), 1006-1019.

Lee, M.J., Chen, F. (2017). Circulating humorous antitobacco videos on social media: Platform *versus* context. *Health Promotion Practice,* 18(2), 184-192. [http://dx.doi.org/10.1177/1524839916677521]

Lee, Y.J., Boden-Albala, B., Larson, E., Wilcox, A., Bakken, S. (2014). Online health information seeking behaviors of Hispanics in New York City: A community-based cross-sectional study. *Journal of Medical Internet Research,* 16(7). [http://dx.doi.org/10.2196/jmir.3499]

Lemire, M., Sicotte, C., Pare, G. (2008). Internet use and the logics of personal empowerment in health. *Health Policy,* 88(1), 130-140.

Lewis, T.L. (2013). A systematic self-certification model for mobile medical apps. *Journal of Medical Internet Research,* 15(4), e89. [http://dx.doi.org/10.2196/jmir.2446]

Lewis, T.L., Wyatt, J.C. (2014). mHealth and mobile medical apps: a framework to assess risk and promote safer use. *Journal of Medical Internet Research,* 16(9), e210. [http://dx.doi.org/10.2196/jmir.3133]

Lewis, T. (2006). Seeking health information on the Internet: lifestyle choice or bad attack of cyberchondria? *Media Culture & Society,* 28, 521-521.

Li, J., Tang, J., Liu, X., Ma, L. (2019). How do users adopt health information from social media? The narrative paradigm perspective. *Health Information Management Journal, 48*(3), 116-126. [http://dx.doi.org/10.1177/1833358318798742]

Li, J., Theng, Y-L., Foo, S. (2015). Predictors of online health information seeking behavior: Changes between 2002 and 2012. *Health Informatics Journal, 22*, 1-11.

Li, Y., Wang, X., Lin, X., Hajli, M. (2018). Seeking and sharing health information on social media: A net valence model and cross-cultural comparison. *Technological Forecasting & Social Change, 126*, 28-40. [http://dx.doi.org/10.1016/j.techfore.2016.07.021]

Lin, N. (2001). *A theory of social structure and action..* Cambridge, UK: Cambridge University Press.

Lin, W-Y., Zhang, X., Song, H., Omori, K. (2016). Health information seeking in the Web 2.0 age: Trust in social media, uncertainty reduction, and self-disclosure. *Computers in Human Behavior, 56*, 289-294.

Lorence, D.P., Park, H., Fox, S. (2006). Racial disparities in health information access: Resilience of the digital divide. *Journal of Medical Systems, 30*, 241-249.

Lucivero, F., Jongsma, K.R. (2018). A mobile revolution for healthcare? Setting the agenda for bioethics. *Journal of Medical Ethics, 44*(10), 685-689.

Lupton, D. (2016). Digital health technologies and digital data: new ways of monitoring, measuring and commodifying human embodiment, health and illness. In: Xavier Olleros, F., Zhegu, M., (Eds.), *Research Handbook on Digital Transformations*Northampton: Edward Elgar.

Lurie, J (2003). Error-free software is in reach, but is anyone reaching? http://www.devx.com/enterprise/Article/16687

Lustria, M.L., Smith, S.A., Hinnant, C. (2011). Exploring digital divides: examination of health technology use, health information seeking, communication and personal health management. *Health Informatics Journal, 17*, 224-243.

Lutz, C. (2016). A social milieu approach to the online participation divides in Germany. *Social Media + Society, 2*(1), 1-14.

Maarse, H., Paulus, A. (2003). Has solidarity survived? A comparative analysis of the effect of social health insurance reform in four European countries. *Journal of Health Politics, Policy and Law, 28*(4), 585-614.

Mackenbach, J. (2012). The persistence of health inequalities in modern welfare states: the explanation of paradox. *Social Science & Medicine, 75*(4), 761-769.

Mackenbach, J.P., Stirbu, I., Roskam, A.J.R., Schaap, M.M., Menvielle, G., Leinsalu, M., Kunst, A.E. (2008). Socioeconomic inequalities in health in 22 European countries. *New England journal of medicine, 358*(23), 2468-2481.

Magnezi, R., Grosberg, D., Novikov, I., Ziv, A., Shani, M., Freedman, L.S. (2015). Characteristics of patients seeking health information online *via* social health networks *versus* general Internet sites: A comparative study. *Informatics for Health and Social Care, 40*(2), 125-138. [http://dx.doi.org/10.3109/17538157.2013.879147]

Malvey, D., Slovensky, D.J. (2014). *mHealth: transforming healthcare.* Springer.New York:

Manchaiah, V., Pyykkő, I., Pyykkő, N. (2020). The use of the internet and social media by individuals with

Ménière's disease: an exploratory survey of finnish Ménière federation members. *Journal of International Advanced Otology, 16*(1), 13-17.

Manhattan Research. (2012). *Cybercitizen Health: Europe.* http://www.ihealthbeat.org/data-points /2012/what-percentage-of-eu-internet-users-have-pursued-healthrelated-activities-online.aspx#ixzz2Mrm5 uTVc

Mano, R. (2018). Online and virtual health information uses, health empowerment and health risks. *Journal of Community Preventive Medicine, 1*(2), 1-7.

Mano, R., Mesch, G., Tsamir, Y. (2009). *Health electronic services in Israel and inequality, Report..* Tel Aviv: Maccabi Health Services.

Mano, R (2019). Mobile health applications and the self-management of cancer: A gendered approach. *Open Journal of Preventive Medicine, 9*, 21-32.

Mano, R. (2014). Social media and online health services: A health empowerment perspective to online health information. *Computers in Human Behavior, 3*, 404-412.

Mano, R. (2015). Online health information, situational effects and health changes among e-patients in Israel: A "push / pull" perspective. *Health Expect., 18*(6), 2489-2500.

Mano, R. (2016). Chronic illness, online health information and online health services. *International Journal of Hospital Administration, 5*(4), 55-60.
[http://dx.doi.org/10.5430/jha.v5n4p55]

Mano, R. (2016). Online health information and health changes: A gender approach to technology and health empowerment among Jewish women in Israel. *Journal of Community Medicine & Public Health Care, 3*, 023.

Mano, R. (2018). Use of mobile health applications and the self-management of chronic disease. *Diversity and equality in health care, 15*(5), 5-25.

Mano, R.G., Mesch, Y.Tsamir (2009). *Inequalities in health care and health services, Unpublished Report, Maccabi Health Insurance Organization, Tel Aviv.*

Mantovani, E, Guihen Barry, B, Quinn, P, Habbig, A-K, De Hert, P (2013). eHealth to mHealth. A journey precariously dependent upon apps? *European Journal of ePractice, 21*, 48-66.

Marler, W. (2018). Mobile phones and inequality: Findings, trends, and future directions. *New Media & Society, 20*(9), 3498-3520.

Marmor, T., Wendt, C. (2011). *Reforming healthcare systems.* UK: Edward Elgar Publishing.

Marmor, T., Wendt, C. (2012). Conceptual frameworks for comparing healthcare politics and policy. *Health Policy, 107*(1), 11-20.

Marston, H.R., Smith, S.T. (2013). Understanding the digital game classification system: a review of the current classification system and its implications for use within games for health. In: Holzinger, A., Ziefle, M., Hitz, M., Debevc, M., (Eds.), (pp. 314-331). Berlin: Springer.

Marton, C., Choo, C.W. (2012). A review of theoretical models of health information seeking on the web. *Journal of Documentation.*

Matthys, J., Elwyn, G., Van Nuland, M., Van Maele, G., De Sutter, A. (2009). Patients' ideas, concerns, and

expectations (ICE) in general practice: impact on prescribing. *British Journal of General Practice, 59*(558), 29-36.
[http://dx.doi.org/10.3399/bjgp09X394833]

Mattke, S., Klautzer, L., Mengistu, T., Garnett, J., Hu, J., Wu, H. (2012). *Health and well-being in the home: A global analysis of needs, expectations, and priorities for Home health care technology..* Rand, California Press.

May, C., Finch, T. (2009). Implementing, Embedding, and Integrating Practices: An Outline of Normalization Process Theory. *Sociology,   43*(3), 535-554.

Mccoll-Kennedy, J.R., Snyder, H., Elg, M., Witell, L., Helkkula, A., Hogan, S.J., Anderson, L. (2017). The changing role of the health care customer: Review, synthesis and research agenda. Journal of Service. *Management, 28*(1), 2-33.
[http://dx.doi.org/10.1108/josm-01-2016-0018]

McFarlane,   B   (2014).   *FDA   regulation   ofmobile   medical   apps.*   https://www.namsa.com/wp-content/uploads/2015/10/WP-FDA-Regulation-of-Mobile-Medical-Apps-7-7-2014.pdf

McKinstry, B. (1992). Paternalism and the doctor-patient relationship in general practice. *Br. J. Gen. Pract., 42*, 340-342.

McPherson, K. (1989). International differences in medical care practices. *Health care financing review,* 9-20.

Medical Device and Diagnosis Industry. (2015). *Consumer mHealth app or regulated medical device?.*
http://www.mddionline.com/blog/devicetalk/consumer-mhealth-app-or-regulated-medical-device-03-04-15

Meldrum, S., Savarimuthu, B.T.R., Licorish, S., Tahir, A., Bosu, M., Jayakaran, P. (2017). Is knee pain information on YouTube videos perceived to be helpful? An analysis of user comments and implications for dissemination on social media. *Digital Health, 3*, 1-18.
[http://dx.doi.org/10.1177/2055207617698908]

Merchant, K. (2012). How men and women differ: gender differences in communication styles, influence tactics, and leadership styles. *CMC Senior Theses, 513.*

Merolli, M., Gray, K., Martin-Sanchez, F. (2013). Health outcomes and related effects of using social media in chronic disease management: A literature review and analysis of affordances. *Journal of Biomedical Informatics, 46*(6), 957-969.
[http://dx.doi.org/10.1016/j.jbi.2013.04.010]

Mesch, G., Talmud, I. (2006). Online friendship formation, communication channels, and social closeness. *International Journal of Internet Sciences, 1*(1), 29-44. Available at: http://www.ijis.net/

Mesch, G., Talmud, I. (2011). Ethnic differences in internet access: the role of occupation and exposure to information. *Communication & Society, 14*(4).

Mesch, G.S. (2016). Ethnic origin and access to electronic health services. *Health Informatics Journal, 22*(4), 791-803.

Mesch, G.S., Talmud, I. (2007). Editorial Comment: e-Relationships–the blurring and reconfiguration of offline and online social boundaries. *Information, Communication & Society, 10*(5), 585-589.

Mesch, G., Talmud, I. (2006). The quality of online and offline relationships: The role of multiplexity and

duration of social relationships. *The Information Society, 22*(3), 137-148.
[http://dx.doi.org/10.1080/01972240600677805]

Mesch, G., Mano, R., Tsamir, Y. (2012). Minority status and the search for health information online: a test of the social diversification hypothesis. *Social Science & Medicine, 75*(5), 854-858.

Mesch, G.S. (2009). Parental mediation, online activities, and cyberbullying. *CyberPsychology & Behavior, 12*(4), 387-393.
[http://dx.doi.org/10.1089/cpb.2009.0068]

Mesch, G.S. (2012). Minority status and the use of computer-mediated communication: A test of the social diversification hypothesis. *Communication Research, 39*(3), 317-337.
[http://dx.doi.org/10.1177/0093650211398865]

Mesch, G.S. Perceptions of risk, lifestyle activities, and fear of crime. *Deviant Behavior, 21*(1), 47-62.
[http://dx.doi.org/10.1080/016396200266379]

Mesch, G.S., Beker, G. (2010). Are norms of disclosure of online and offline personal information associated with the disclosure of personal information online? *Human Communication Research, 36*, 570-592.
[http://dx.doi.org/10.1111/j.1468-2958.2010.01389.x]

Mesny, A. (2009). What do 'we' know that 'they' don't? Sociologists' *versus* nonsociologists' knowledge. *Canadian   Journal   of   Sociology,   34,   671-*695.https://journals.library.ualberta.ca/cjs/index.php/cjs/article/view/6313

Micheli, M., Lutz, C., Büchi, M. (2018). Digital footprints: An emerging dimension of digital inequality. *Journal of Information. Communication and Ethics in Society, 16*(3), 242-251.

Mikulic, M. (2020). *Statista: Mobile medical apps market size worldwide 2017 and 2025.*

Millenson, M.L., Baldwin, J.L., Zipperer, L., Singh, H. (2018). Beyond Dr. Google: the evidence on consumer-facing digital tools for diagnosis. *Diagnosis (Berl.), 5*(3), 95-105.
[http://dx.doi.org/10.1515/dx-2018-0009]

Miller, C. A., Guidry, J. P., Fuemmeler, B. F. (2019). Breast Cancer Voices on Pinterest: Raising Awareness or Just an Inspirational Image? *Health Education & Behavior, 46*(2_suppl), 49S-58S.

Mo, P.K.H., Coulson, N.S. (2014). Are online support groups always beneficial?: A qualitative exploration of the empowering and disempowering processes of participation within HIV/AIDS-related online support groups. *International Journal of Nursing Studies, 51*, 983-993.

Moran, M. (1999). *Governing the health care state: a comparative study of the United Kingdom, the United States, and Germany.* UK: Manchester University Press.

Moretti, F.A., Barsottini, C. (2017). Support, attention and distant guidance for chronic pain patients: Case report. *Revista Dor, 18*, 85-87.

Mossialos, E. (1997). Citizens' views on health care systems in the 15 member states of the European Union. *Health economics, 6*(2), 109-116.

Mossialos, E., Dixon, A., Kutzin, J., Figueras, J. (2002). Funding health care: options for Europe. *European Observatory on Health Care Systems Series.* Buckingham, Philadelphia: Open University Press.

Murero, M., Rice, R. (2006). *The Internet and health care..* New Jersey: LEA & Associates.

Musiat, P., Goldstone, P., Tarrier, N. (2014). Understanding the acceptability of e-mental health—attitudes and expectations towards computerised self-help treatments for mental health problems. *BMC Psychiatry, 14*(1), 109.
[http://dx.doi.org/10.1186/1471-244x-14-109]

Napoli, P., Obar, J. (2014). The emerging mobile Internet underclass: A critique of mobile Internet access. *The Information Society, 30*(5), 323-334.

National Telecommunications and Information Administration. (2000). *Falling through the Net II: Toward digital inclusion.*http://www.ntia.doc.gov/ntiahome/fttn00/contents00.html

National Telecommunications and Information Administration. (2002). *A nation online: how Americans are expanding their use of the Internet.*http://www.ntia.doc.gov/ntiahome/dn/index.html

Nelson, R. (2017). "Informatics: Empowering ePatients to Drive Healthcare Reform - Part II" OJIN. *The Online Journal of Issues in Nursing, 22*(3), 9.

Neuner, J., Fedders, M., Caravella, M., Bradford, L., Schapira, M. (2015). Meaningful use and the patient portal: patient enrollment, use, and satisfaction with patient portals at a later-adopting center. *American Journal of Medical Quality, 30*(2), 105-113.

Neves, B.B., Fonseca, J.R., Amaro, F., Pasqualotti, A. (2018). Social capital and Internet use in an age-comparative perspective with a focus on later life. *PLoS One, 13*(2)

Newlands, G., Lutz, C., Fieseler, C. (2018). Collective action and provider classification in the sharing economy. *New Technology, Work and Employment, 33*(3), 250-267.

Newman, M.W., Lauterbach, D., Munson, S.A., Resnick, P., Morris, M.E. (2011). It's not that I don't have problems, I'm just not putting them on Facebook. *Proceedings of the ACM 2011 Conference on Computer-Supported Cooperative Work,* New York, NYACM. 341-350. nl/Over-KNMG/About-KNMG/Ne-s-English/152830/Medical-App-Checker-a-Guide-to-assessing-Mobile-Medical-Apps.htm

Noble, S.U. (2018). *Algorithms of oppression: How search engines reinforce racism..* New York: NYU Press.

Nolte, E., McKee, C.M. (2008). Measuring the health of nations: updating an earlier analysis. *Health affairs, 27*(1), 58-71.

Nolte, E., McKee, M. (2011). Variations in amenable mortality—trends in 16 high-income nations. *Health Policy, 103*(1), 47-52.

Norris, P. (2001). *Digital divide: Civic engagement, information poverty, and the Internet worldwide..* Cambridge, MA: Cambridge University Press.

OECD. (1999). *Improving Evaluation Practices: Best Practice Guidelines for Evaluation and Background Paper.* Paris, France.

Office of Evaluation and Strategic Planning. (1997). New York.

Oh, H.J., Lauckner, C., Boehmer, J., Fewins-Bliss, R., Li, K. (2013). Facebooking for health: An examination into the solicitation and effects of health-related social support on social networking sites. *Computers in Human Behavior, 29*(5), 2072-2080.
[http://dx.doi.org/10.1016/j.chb.2013.04.017]

Okun, S., Caligan, C. (2018). The Evolving ePatient. In: Nelson, R., Staggers, N., (Eds.), *Health Informatics: An Interprofessional Approach.* (2nd ed., pp. 204-219). St Louis: Elsevier.

Ontario Ministry of Health and Long-Term Care. (2007). Introduction to evaluation health promotion programs.*Public Health Branch In: The Health Communication Unit at the Centre for Health Promotion.*

OpenmHealth. (2019). *Want To Use Mobile Health Data AND Have It To Make Sense?.*

Orben, A., Przybylski, A.K. (2019). The association between adolescent wellbeing and digital technology use. *Nature Human Behaviour, 3*, 173-182.

Organisation for Economic Co-operation and Development. (1990). *Health care systems in transition: the search for efficiency.*

Organisation for Economic Co-operation and Development. Washington, DC: OECD Publications and Information Centre.

Ostrom, A.L., Parasuraman, A., Bowen, D.E., Patricio, L., Voss, C.A. (2015). Service research priorities in a rapidly changing context. *Journal of Service Research, 18*(2), 127-159. [http://dx.doi.org/10.1177/1094670515576315]

Parker, L., Bero, L., Gillies, D., Raven, M., Mintzes, B., Jureidini, J., Grundy, Q. (2018). Mental health messages in prominent mental health apps. *Annals of Family Medicine, 16*(4), 338-342. https://doi-org.ezproxy.haifa.ac.il/10.1370/afm.2260

Peacock, S., Reddy, A., Leveille, S.G., Walker, J., Payne, T.H., Oster, N.V., Elmore, J.G. (2017). Patient portals and personal health information online: perception, access, and use by US adults. *Journal of the American Medical Informatics Association, 24*(e1), e173-e177.

Pearce, K., Rice, R. (2013). Digital divides from access to activities: Comparing mobile and personal computer Internet users. *Journal of Communication, 63*(4), 721-744.

Pena-Purcell, N. (2008). Hispanics' use of Internet health information: An exploratory study. *Journal Medical Library Association, 96*(2), 101-107.

Fox, S., Durgan, M. (2013). *Tracking for health.* Pew Research Center. http://www.pewinternet.org/2013/01/28/tracking-for-health-2/

Pew Research Center. (2013). *Health fact sheet: Highlights of the Pew Internet Project's research related to health and health care.*http://www. pewinternet.org/fact-sheets/health-fact-sheet/

Internet/broadband fact sheet. Washington, DC: Pew Research Center: Internet & Technology. http://www.pewinternet.org/fact-sheet/ internet-broadband/

Pfizer, U.K. (2011). *Dear doctor letter: "Pfizer rheumatology calculator" iPhone/android applica- tion — important information.*http://www.pharma-mkting.com/images/Pfizer_Rheum_BugLetter.pdf

Pierson, P. (2002). Coping with permanent austerity: welfare state restructuring in affluent democracies. *Revue française de sociologie,* 369-406.

Potts, H.W., Wyatt, J.C. (2002). Survey of doctors' experience of patients using the internet. *Journal of Medical Internet Research, 4*(1), e5.

Pousti, H., Urquhart, C., Linger, H. (2014). Exploring the role of social media in chronic care management: A sociomaterial approach. *Working Conference on Information Systems and Organizations* (pp. 163-185). Berlin, Heidelberg: Springer.

Power, J. M., Phelan, S., Hatley, K., Brannen, A., Muñoz-Christian, K., Legato, M., Tate, D. F. (2019). Engagement and weight loss in a web and mobile program for low-income postpartum women: Fit moms/mamás activas. *Health Education & Behavior,* *46*(2_suppl), 114S-123S.

Prainsack, B. (2014). The powers of participatory medicine. *PLOS Biology,* *12*(4), e1001837.

Purcell, K., Fox, S. (2010). Chronic disease and the Internet. *Pew and American Life Project.*http://www.pewinternet.org/Reports/2010/Chronic-Disease.aspx

PWC. (2012). *Emerging mHealth: Paths for growth.*www.pwc.com/mhealth

Quinn, P. (2013). Medical apps and accountability – where can the patient/consumer find protec- tion? *European Journal of Health Law.Fourth Conference on European Health Law, Book of Abstracts.*

Ragnedda, M., Muschert, G.W. (2013). *The digital divide: The internet and social inequality in international perspective.* UK: Routledge. https://ebookcentral.proquest.com

Raijman, R. (2016). *South African Jews in Israel: Assimilation in multigenerational perspective.* Nebraska, United States: University of Nebraska Press.

Rains, S.A. (2007). Perceptions of traditional information sources and use of the World Wide Web to seek health information. *Journal of Health Communication: International Perspectives,* *12*, 667-680.

Rasmussen, E.E., LaFreniere, Jenna R., Norman, Mary S., Kimball, Thomas G. Narissra Punyanunt-Carter. (2020). The serially mediated relationship between emerging adults' social media use and mental well-being. *Computers in Human Behavior,* *102*, 206-213.

Reading, J. M., Buhr, K. J., Stuckey, H. L. (2019). Social experiences of adults using online support forums to lose weight: A qualitative content analysis. *Health Education & Behavior,* *46*(2_suppl), 129S-133S.

Rechel, B. (2019). A Framework for Health System Comparisons: The Health Systems in Transition (HiT) Series of the European Observatory on Health Systems and Policies. In: Adrian Levy, A., Goring, S., Gatsonis, C., Sobolev, B., Ginneken, E.V., (Eds.), *Health Services Evaluation, Health Services Research* (pp. 279-296). New York, NY: Springer.

Reczek, C., Umberson, D. (2012). Gender, health behavior, and intimate relationships: Lesbian, gay, and straight contexts. *Social Science & Medicine,* *74*(11), 1783-1790. [http://dx.doi.org/10.1016/j.socscimed.2011.11.011]

Reibling, N., Wendt, C. (2011). Regulating patients' access to healthcare services. *International Journal of Public and Private Healthcare Management and Economics (IJPPHME),* *1*(2), 1-16. [IJPPHME].

Renahy, E., Parizot, I., Chauvin, P. (2008). Health information seeking on the internet: A double-divide? Results from a representative survey in the Paris metropolitan area, France, 2005-2006. *BMC Public Health,* 1-10.

Research2Guidance. (2016). *mHealth app developer economics.* http:// research2guidance.com/r2g/r2g-mHealth-App-Developer-Economics-2016.pdf

Rice, R. (2006). Influences, usage and outcomes of internet health information searching: Multivariate results from the Pew surveys. *International Journal of Medical Informatics,* *75*(1), 8-28.

Riggare, S., Höglund, P.J., Forsberg, H.H., Eftimovska, E., Svenningsson, P., Hägglund, M. (2017). Patients are doing it for themselves: A survey on disease-specific knowledge acquisition among people with Parkinson's disease in Sweden. *Health Informatics Journal,* *25*(1), 91-105.
[http://dx.doi.org/10.1177/1460458217704248]

Riley, W. T., Oh, A., Aklin, W. M., Wolff-Hughes, D. L. (2019). National institutes of health support of digital health behavior research. *Health Education & Behavior,* *46*(2_suppl), 12S-19S.

Risk, A., Petersen, C. (2002). Health information on the internet: quality issues and international initiatives. *JAMA,* *87*(20), 2713-5.

Rissel, C. (1993). Empowerment: The holy grail of health promotion? *Health Promotion International,* *9*(1), 39-47.

Robinson, J.R., Davis, S.E., Cronin, R.M., Jackson, G.P. (2016). Use of a patient portal during hospital admissions to surgical services. *AMIA Annual Symposium Proceedings,* 1967-1976.

Robinson, L., Cotten, S., Ono, H., QuanHaase, A., Mesch, G., Chen, W., Stern, M. (2015). Digital inequalities and why they matter. *Information, Communication & Society,* *18*(5), 569-582.

Roeser, S. (2018). *Risk, technology, and moral emotions..* New York, NY: Routledge.

Rogers, E.S., Chamberlin, J., Ellison, M.L., Crean, T. (1997). A consumer-constructed scale to measure empowerment among users of mental health services. *Psychiatric Services,* *48*(8), 1042-1047.

Ronfenbrenner, Urie (1979). *The Ecology of Human Development: Experiments by Nature and Design.* Cambridge, MA: Harvard University Press.

Rosenberg, D., Mano, R., Mesch, G. (2017). They have needs, they have goals: using communication theories to explain health-related social media use and health behavior change. *MOJ Public Health,* *6*(2), 00163.
[http://dx.doi.org/10.15406/mojph.2017.06.00163]

Rosenberg, D., Mano, R., Mesh, G. (2019). Absolute monopoly", "areas of control" or "democracy"? Examining gender differences in health participation on social media. *Computers in Human Behavior.*

Rosser, B.A., Eccleston, C. (2011). Smartphone applications for pain management. *Journal of Telemedicine and Telecare,* *17*(6), 308-312.
[http://dx.doi.org/10.1258/jtt.2011.101102]

Rozenblum, R., Greaves, F., Bates, D.W. (2017). The role of social media around patient experience and engagement. *BMJ Quality & Safety,* *26*(10), 845-848.

Rübsamen, K, Sakellariou, S (2015). *Mobile health apps: are they a regulated medical device?.*
http://www.whitecase.com/publications/article/mobile-health-apps-are-they-regulated-medical-device

Salmon, P., Hall, G.K. (2003). Patient empowerment and control: a psychological discourse in the service of medicine. *Social Science & Medicine,* *57*(10), 1969-1980.

Saltman, R.B. (1997). Equity and distributive justice in European health care reform. *International Journal of Health Services,* *27*(3), 443-453.

Scalvini, S., Baratti, D., Assoni, G., Zanardini, M., Comini, L., Bernocchi, P. (2013). Information and communication technology in chronic diseases: a patient's opportunity. *Journal of Medicine and the Person,* *12*(3), 1-5.

Scanfeld, D., Scanfeld, V., Larson, E.L. (2010). Dissemination of health information through social networks: Twitter and antibiotics. *American Journal of Infection Control, 38*(3), 182-188.
[http://dx.doi.org/10.1016/j.ajic.2009.11.004]

Scheerder, A., Van Deursen, A., Van Dijk, J. (2017). Determinants of Internet skills, uses and outcomes. A systematic review of the secondand thirdlevel digital divide. *Telematics and Informatics, 34*(8), 1607-1624.

Scheiber, G. J. (1987). *Financing and delivering health care: a comparative analysis of OECD countries.* Paris, France: Organisation for Economic Co-operation and Development.

Schiavo, R. (2007). *Health communication: from theory to practice..* San Francisco: Jossey-Bass.

Schieber, G.J., Poullier, J.P. (1989). Overview of international comparisons of health care expenditures. *Health care financing review,* (Suppl.), 1.

Schnall, R., Higgins, T., Brown, W., Carballo-Dieguez, A., Bakken, S. (2015). Trust, perceived risk, perceived ease of use and perceived usefulness as factors related to mHealth technology use. *Studies in Health Technology and Informatics, 216,* 467-471.
[http://dx.doi.org/10.3233/978-1-61499-564-7-467]

Schrecker, T., Bambra, C. (2015). *How Politics Makes Us Sick: Neoliberal Epidemics.* London: Palgrave Macmillan.

Ralph, S., Caldas, A., Dutton, W., Mesch, G. (2008). Patterns of Information Search and Access on the World Wide Web: Democratizing Expertise or Creating New Hierarchies? *Journal of Computer Mediated Communication, 13*(4), 769-793.

Schulze, E-D. (2005). *Plant Ecology..* Berlin: Springer.

Schuster, L., Drennan, J., Lings, I.N. (2013). Consumer acceptance of m-wellbeing services: A social marketing perspective. *European Journal of Marketing, 47*(9), 1439-1457.
[http://dx.doi.org/10.1108/ejm-10-2011-0556]

Sebastian, J., Richards, D. (2017). Changing stigmatizing attitudes to mental health *via* education and contact with embodied conversational agents. *Computers in Human Behavior, 73,* 479-488.
[http://dx.doi.org/10.1016/j.chb.2017.03.071]

Seth, M.N., Grant-Harrington, N. (2012). *eHealth applications: Promising strategies for behavior change.* UK: Routledge.

Shim, M., Kelly, B., Hornik, R. (2006). Cancer information scanning and seeking behavior associated with knowledge, lifestyle choices and screening. *Journal of Health Communication, 1,* 157-172.

Sillence, E, Briggs, P., Harris, P. R. (2007). How do patients evaluate and make use of online health information? *Social Science & Medicine, 64,* 1853-1862.

Silver, R.A., Subramaniam, C., Stylianou, A. (2020). The Impact of Portal Satisfaction on Portal Use and Health-Seeking Behavior: Structural Equation Analysis. *Journal of Medical Internet Research,* 16260.

Singleton, A., Abeles, P., Smith, I.C. (2016). Online social networking and psychological experiences: The perceptions of young people with mental health difficulties. *Computers in Human Behavior, 61,* 394-403.

[http://dx.doi.org/10.1016/j.chb.2016.03.011]

Siu, A.L., Mittman, B.S. (1992). Implementing outcomes and effectiveness research in health care.*The Baxter Health Policy Review.* Health Administration Press.

Smailhodzic, E., Attema, S. (2016). Self-determination theory as an explaining mechanism for the effects of patient's social media use. *ICIS '16 Proceedings of the International Conference on Information Systems.* Dublin, Ireland: AIS.

Smith, B.J., Tang, K.C., Nutbeam, D. (2006). *WHO Health Promotion Glossary: new terms Health Promotion International,* *21*(4)

Smith, P.C., Anell, A., Busse, R., Crivelli, L., Healy, J., Lindahl, A.K. (2012). Leadership and governance in seven developed health systems. *Health Policy,* *106*(1), 37-49.

Smith, P.C., Mossialos, E., Leatherman, S., Papanicolas, I. (2009). *Performance measurement for health system improvement: experiences, challenges and prospects..* UK: Cambridge University Press.

Smith, PC., Busse, R. (2009). Targets and performance measurement. In: Smith, PC., Mossialos, E., Papanicolas, I., Leatherman, S., (Eds.), *Performance Measurement for Health System Improvement: Experiences, Challenges and Prospects.* Cambridge: Cambridge University Press.

Smock, A.D., Ellison, N.B., Lampe, C., Wohn, D.Y. (2011). Facebook as a toolkit: A uses and gratification approach to unbundling feature use. *Computers in Human Behavior,* *27*, 2322-2329. [http://dx.doi.org/10.1016/j.chb.2011.07.011]

Sorenson, C., Drummond, M. (2016). Improving medical device regulation: the United States and Europe in perspective. *Milbank Quarterly,* *92*(1), 145-150.

Srinivasan, R., Fish, A. (2017). *After the Internet..* Cambridge: Polity Press.

Stallman, H.M., Ohan, J.L., Chiera, B. (2018). The role of social support, being present and selfkindness in university student wellbeing. *British Journal of Guidance & Counselling,* *46*(4), 365-374. b

Stefanescu, E.D.N., Bilcan, F.R., Ifrim, A.M. (2019). Analysing the consumer behaviour of online health services. *Academic Journal of Economic Studies,* *5*(3), 126-131.

Steinmo, S., Watts, J. (1995). It's the institutions, stupid! Why comprehensive national health insurance always fails in America. *Journal of Health Politics, Policy and Law,* *20*(2), 329-372.

Stellefson, M., Hanik, B., Chaney, B., Chaney, D., Tennant, B., Chavarria, E.A. (2011). eHealth literacy among college students: A systematic review with implications for eHealth education. *Journal of Medical Internet Research,* *13*(4), e102. [http://dx.doi.org/10.2196/jmir.1703]

Stokols, D. (1996). Translating social ecological theory into guidelines for community health promotion. *American Journal of Health Promotion,* *10*, 282-298. [http://dx.doi.org/10.4278/0890-1171-10.4.282]

Stokols, D. (1992). Establishing and maintaining healthy environments: toward a social ecology of health promotion. *American Psychologist,* *47*, 6-22. [http://dx.doi.org/10.1037/0003-066x.47.1.6]

Streiner, D.L., Geoffrey, N.R. (2008). *Health measurement scales: a practical guide to their development and use.* Oxford: Oxford University Press.

Stuckler, D., Basu, S. (2013). *The body economic: why austerity kills. Recessions, budget battles, and the politics of life and death.* New York, NY: Basic Books.

Su, R., Tay, L., Diener, E. (2014). The Development and Validation of the Comprehensive Inventory of Thriving (CIT) and the Brief Inventory of Thriving (BIT). *Applied Psychology. Health and Well□Being, 6*(3), 251-271.

Sundmacher, L., Busse, R. (2011). The impact of physician supply on avoidable cancer deaths in Germany. A spatial analysis. *Health Policy, 103*(1), 53-62.

Gümüş, R., Sönmez, Y. (2020). Quality of online communication tools at hospitals and their effects on health service consumers' preferences. *International Journal of Healthcare Management, 13*(1), 35-44. [http://dx.doi.org/10.1080/20479700.2018.1470816]

Sweeney, L. (2000). Uniqueness of simple demographics in the U.S. *Population.* Pittsburgh.

Szasz, T.S., Hollender, M.H. (1956). A Contribution to the Philosophy of Medicine: The Basic Models of the Doctor-Patient Relationship. *Archives of Internal Medicine, 97*(5), 585-592.

Taiminen, H., Saraniemi, S. (2018). Acceptance of Online Health Services for Self-Help in the Context of Mental Health: Understanding Young Adults' Experiences. *Journal of Technology in Human Services, 36*(2/3), 125-139.https://doi-org.ezproxy.haifa.ac.il/10.1080/15228835.2018.1426081

Tang, W., Ren, J., Zhang, Y. (2019). Enabling trusted and privacy-preserving healthcare services in social media health networks. *IEEE Transactions on Multimedia, 21*(3), 579-590. https://doi-org.ezproxy. haifa.ac.il/10.1109/TMM.2018.2889934

Tavares, J., Oliveira, T. (2016). Electronic health record patient portal adoption by health care consumers: an acceptance model and survey. *Journal of Medical Internet Research, 18*(3), e49.

Taylor, T.E. (2015). The markers of wellbeing: A basis for a theory-neutral approach. *International Journal of Wellbeing, 5*(2), 75-90. [http://dx.doi.org/10.5502/ijw.v5i2.5]

Tene, O, Polonetsky, J (2013). Big data for all: privacy and user control in the age of analytics. *Northwestern Journal of Technology and Intellectual Property, 11*(5), xxvii-274.

Terrasse, M.Gorin, Sisti, D. (2019). Social Media, e-Health, and Medical Ethics. *Hastings Center Report, 49*(1), 24-33.

Thackeray, R., Crookston, B.T., West, J.H. (2013). Correlates of health-related social media use among adults. *Journal of Medical Internet Research, 15*(1), e21. [http://dx.doi.org/10.2196/jmir.2297]

Thaler, R., Sunstein, C. (2008). *Nudge: improving decisions about health, wealth, and happiness..* New Haven, CT: Yale University Press.

Thelwall, M., Wilkinson, D., Uppal, S. (2009). Data mining emotion in social network communication: Gender differences in MySpace. *Journal of the American Society for Information Science and Technology Banner, 61*(1), 190-199. [http://dx.doi.org/10.1002/asi.21180]

Thompson, BM, Brodsky, I (2013). Should the FDA regulate mobile medical apps? *BMJ, 347*, f5211-f5211.

Thomson, S., Foubister, T., Mossialos, E. (2009). Financing health care in the European Union: challenges and policy responses. *World Health Organization*Regional Office for Europe.

Tian, K., Sautter, P., Fisher, D., Fischbach, S., Luna-Nevarez, C., Boberg, K. (2014). Transforming health care: Empowering therapeutic communities through technology-enhanced narratives. *Journal of Consumer Research, 41*(2), 237-260.
[http://dx.doi.org/10.1086/676311]

TIM. (2010). *Patterns of use of Internet in Israel.* http://www.pc.co.il/?p=25351

Torabi, S., Beznosov, K. (2016). Sharing health information on facebook: practices, preferences, and risk perceptions of North American users. *Twelfth Symposium on Usable Privacy and Security ({SOUPS} 2016),* 301-320.

Tsetsi, E., Rains, S. (2017). Smartphone Internet access and use: Extending the digital divide and usage gap. *Mobile Media & Communication, 5*(3), 239-255.

Tuohy, C.H. (1999). *Accidental logics: The dynamics of change in the health care arena in the United States, Britain, and Canada..* UK: Oxford University Press.

Tuohy, C.H. (2003). Agency, contract, and governance: shifting shapes of accountability in the health care arena. *Journal of Health Politics, Policy and Law, 28*(2-3), 195-216.

Turjeman, H., Mesch, G., Fishman, G. (2008). The effect of acculturation on depressive moods: Immigrant boys and girls during their transition from late adolescence to early adulthood. *International Journal of Psychology, 43*(1), 32-44.
[http://dx.doi.org/10.1080/00207590701804362]

Tustin, N. (2010). The role of patient satisfaction in online health information seeking. *Journal of Health Communication, 15*(1), 3-17.

U.S. Centres for Disease Control and Prevention (CDC). (1999). *Framework for Program Evaluation in Public Health.*http://www.cdc.gov/eval/over.htm

U.S. Department of Health and Human Services. (1997). *Administration on Children, Youth, and Families (ACYF).*The Program Manager's Guide to Evaluation.

UNDP. (1997). *Results-Oriented Monitoring and Evaluation: A Handbook for Programme Managers.* New York.

UNICEF. (1991). *A UNICEF Guide for Monitoring and Evaluation: Making a Difference?* New York: Evaluation Office.

UNICEF. (2004). *Evaluation Reports Standards.*

United States Congress. (1938). *Federal Food.* Drug, and Cosmetic Act. https://www.epw.senate.gov/ FDA_001.pdf

United States Congress. (1976). *Medical device amendment.* https://www.congress.gov/bill/94th-congress/house-bill/11124

US Food and Drugs Administration. (2013). *Mobile medical Applications.* http://www.gpo.gov/fdsys /pkg/FR-2013-09-25/pdf/2013-23293.pdf

US Food and Drugs Administration. (2013). *23 and Me, Inc.* http://www.fda.gov /ICECI/ EnforcementActions/WarningLetters/2013/ucm376296.htm

US Food and Drugs Administration. (2015). Mobile medical applications. http://www.fda.gov/downloads/ MedicalDevices/DeviceRegulationandGuidance/GuidanceDocuments/UCM263366.pdf

US Food and Drugs Administration. (2015). *Medical device data systems, medical image storage devices, and medical image communications devices.*http://www.fda.gov/downloads/MedicalDevices/ DeviceRegulationandGuidance/GuidanceDocuments/UCM401996.pdf

US Food and Drugs Administration. (2016). *Examples of mobile apps for which the fda will exercise enforcement discretion.*http://www.fda.gov/MedicalDevices/DigitalHealth/MobileMedicalApplications/ucm368744.htm

US Food and Drugs Administration. (2016). *General wellness: policy for low risk devices.* http://www.fda.gov/downloads/MedicalDevices/DeviceRegulationandGuidance/GuidanceDocuments/UCM4 29674.pdf?source=govdelivery&utm_medium=email&utm_source=govdelivery

USAID Performance Monitoring and Evaluation Tips, TIPS # 3: Preparing an Evaluation Scope of work.

Van der Kleij, R, Kasteleyn, MJ, Meijer, E, Meijer, E, Bonten, T.N, Houwink, E.J.F, Teichert, M., Van, Luenen S., Vedanthan, R., Evers, A., Car, J., Pinnock, H., Chavannes, N.H. (2019). SERIES: eHealth in primary care. Part 1: Concepts, conditions and challenges. *European Journal of General Practice, 25*(4), 179-189. [http://dx.doi.org/10.1080/13814788.2019.1658190]

Van Deursen, A., Van Dijk, J. (2010). Internet skills and the digital divide. *New Media & Society, 13*(6), 893-911. [http://dx.doi.org/10.1177/1461444810386774]

Van Deursen, A.J.A.M., Helsper, E.J. (2015). The thirdlevel digital divide: Who benefits most from being online? In: Robinson, L., Cotten, S.R., Schulz, J., Hale, T.M., Williams, A., (Eds.), *Communication and Information Technologies Annual (Studies in Media and Communications)* (Vol. 10, pp. 29-52). Bingley, United Kingdom: Emerald Group Publishing Limited. [http://dx.doi.org/10.1108/S2050-206020150000010002]

Van Deursen, A., Helsper, E. (2018). Collateral benefits of Internet use: Explaining the diverse outcomes of engaging with the Internet. *New Media & Society, 20*(7), 2333-2351.

Van Deursen, A., Van Dijk, J. (2011). Internet skills and the digital divide. *New Media & Society, 13*(6), 893-911.

Van Deursen, A., Van Dijk, J. (2014). The digital divide shifts to differences in usage. *New Media & Society, 16*(3), 507-526.

Van Deursen, A., Van Dijk, J. (2019). The firstlevel digital divide shifts from inequalities in physical access to inequalities in material access. *New Media & Society, 21*(2), 354-375.

van Deursen, A., van Dijk, J.A.G.M., Peters, O. (2010). The older the better: Rethinking Internet skills. *The role of gender, age, education, Internet experience, and hours spent online. Paper presented at the 2010 ICA Conference.*Singapore

Van Deursen, A., Helsper, E., Eynon, R., Van Dijk, J. (2017). The compoundness and sequentiality of digital inequality. *International Journal of Communication, 11*, 452-473.

van Dijk, J.A.G.M. (2005). *The deepening divide.*. London: Sage Publications.

Van Doorslaer, E., Masseria, C., Koolman, X. (2006). Inequalities in access to medical care by income in developed countries. *CMAJ, 174*(2), 177-183.

van Velsen, L., Beaujean, D.J., van Gemert-Pijnen, J.E. (2013). Why mobile health app overload drives us crazy, and how to restore the sanity. *BMC Medical Informatics and Decision Making, 13*(1), 23. [http://dx.doi.org/10.1186/1472-6947-13-23]

Vargo, S.L., Lusch, R.F. (2004). Evolving to a new dominant logic for marketing. *Journal of Marketing, 68*(1), 1-17. [http://dx.doi.org/10.1509/jmkg.68.1.1.24036]

Vaterlaus, J.M., Patten, E.V., Roche, C., Young, J.A. (2015). #Gettinghealthy: The perceived influence of social media on young adult health behaviors. *Computers in Human Behavior, 45*, 151-157. [http://dx.doi.org/10.1016/j.chb.2014.12.013]

Venkatesh, V., Davis, F.D. (2000). A theoretical extension of the technology acceptance model: Four longitudinal field studies. *Management science, 46*(2), 186-204.

Venkatesh, V., Morris, M.G., Davis, G.B., Davis, F.D. (2003). User acceptance of information technology: Toward a unified view. *MIS quarterly,* 425-478.

Vernon, J.A., Trujillo, A., Rosenbaum, S., DeBuono, B. (2007). *Low Health Literacy: Implications for National Health Policy.*https://publichealth.gwu.edu/departments/healthpolicy/CHPR/downloads10_4_07.pdf

Wagner, T.H., Baker, L.C., Bundorf, M.K., Snger, S. (2004). Use of the internet for health information by the chronically ill. *Preventing Chronic Disease, 1*(4), A13.

Waitzkin, H. (1986). Micropolitics of medicine: Theoretical issues.*Medical Anthropology Quarterly, 17*, 134-136.Micropolitics of medicine: Theoretical issues.

Chinitz, D., Preker, A., Wasem, J. (1997). Balancing competition and solidarity in health care financing. In: Saltman, R.B., Figueras, J., Sakellarides, C., (Eds.), *Critical Challenges for Health Care Reform in Europe,* Buckingham: Open University Press.55-77.

Wasserman, I.M., Richmond-Abbott, M. (2005). Gender and the internet: Causes of variation in access, level, and scope of use. *Social Science Quarterly, 86*(1), 252-273.

Wathen, C.N., Harris, R.M. (2007). I try to take care of it myself how rural women search for health information. *Qualitative Health Research, 17*(5), 639-651.

Wei, K.K., Teo, H.H., Chan, H.C., Tan, B.C. (2011). Conceptualizing and testing a social cognitive model of the digital divide. *Information Systems Research, 22*(1), 170-187.

Weller, J.A., Dieckman, N.F., Martin, T., Mertz, C.K., Burns, W.J., Peters, E. (2012). Development and testing of an abbreviated numeracy scale: a rasch analysis approach. *Journal of Behavioral Decision Making, 26*, 198-212. https://doi-org.ezproxy.haifa.ac.il/10.1002/bdm.1751

Wendt, C. (2009). Mapping European healthcare systems: a comparative analysis of financing, service provision and access to healthcare. *Journal of European Social Policy, 19*(5), 432-445.

Wendt, C., Kohl, J. (2010). Translating monetary inputs into health care provision: a comparative analysis of the impact of different modes of public policy. *Journal of Comparative Policy Analysis, 12*(1-2), 11-31.

Wendt, C., Frisina, L., Rothgang, H. (2009). Healthcare system types: a conceptual framework for comparison. *Social Policy & Administration, 43*(1), 70-90.

Wendt, C., Kohl, J., Mischke, M., Pfeifer, M. (2009). How do Europeans perceive their healthcare system? Patterns of satisfaction and preference for state involvement in the field of healthcare. *European Sociological Review, 26*(2), 177-192.

West, R. (2006). Identifying key factors for success in delivery: A report of the Stop Smoking Services Workshop. London: Department of Health.

WHO. (2008). Closing the Gap in a Generation. *Health Equity through Action on the Social Determinants of Health. Final report of the commission on social determinants of health*Geneva: World Health Organization. whqlibdoc.who.int/publications/2008/9789241563703_eng.pdf

WHO. (2016). Global Health Observatory Data. *Healthy Life-Expectancy at Birth.*who.int/gho/mortality_burden_disease/life_tables/hale/en/

WHO: UNFPA. (2004). Programme manager's planning monitoring & evaluation toolkit. *Division for oversight services.*

Wilhelm, M.O., Bekkers, R. (2010). Helping behavior, dispositional empathic concern, and the principle of care. *Social Psychology Quarterly, 73*(1), 11-32.

Willis, K., Elmer, S. (2007). *Society, culture and health: |An introduction to health sociology for nurses.* Melbourne: Oxford University Press.

Wilsford, D. (1994). Path dependency, or why history makes it difficult but not impossible to reform health care systems in a big way. *Journal of public policy, 14*(3), 251-283.

Wired. (2014). *These medical apps have doctors and the FDA worried.*http://www.wired.com/2014/07/medical_apps/

Witte, K., Allen, M. (2000). A meta analysis of fear appeals: implications for effective public health campaigns. *Health Education & Behavior, 27*(5), 591-615.

Wolf, J., Moreau, J., Akilov, O. (2013). Diagnostic inaccuracy of Smartphone applications for melanoma detection. *JAMA Dermatol, 149*(4), 422-426.

Wood, W., Ridgewat, C.L. (2010). Gender: An interdisciplinary perspective. *Social Psychology Quarterly, 73*(4), 334-339.

Wood, Stacy (2002). Prior knowledge and complacency in new product learning. *Journal of Consumer Research, 29*(December), 416-426.

Work", 1996 and "TIPS # 11: The Role of Evaluation in USAID", 1997, Centre for Development Information and Evaluation. http://www.dec.org/usaid_eval/#004

World Health Organization – WHO. (2008). Closing the gap in a generation: Health equality through action on the social determinants of health. *Final Report of the Commission on Social Determinants of Health.* Geneva: WHO.

World Health Organization – WHO. (2009). *Towards the development of a mHealth strategy: A literature review.* Columbia University: World Health Organization & the Earth Institute.

Xiao, N., Sharman, R., Rao, H.R., Upadhyaya, S. (2014). Factors influencing online health information search: An empirical analysis of a national cancer-related survey. *Decision Support Systems, 57*, 417-427. [http://dx.doi.org/10.1016/j.dss.2012.10.047]

Ybarra, M., Suman, M. (2008). Reasons, assessments and actions taken: sex and age differences in the use of Internet health information. *Health Education Research, 23*, 512-521.

Yelton, A. (2013). *Bridging the Digital Divide with Mobile Services..* Chicago: ALA Editions.

Zainuddin, N., Tam, L., McCosker, A. (2016). Serving yourself: Value self-creation in health care service. *Journal of Services Marketing, 30*(6), 586-600. [http://dx.doi.org/10.1108/jsm-02-2016-0075]

Zhang, N.J., Terry, A., McHorney, C.A. (2014). Impact of health literacy on medication adherence: a systematic review and meta analysis. *Annals of Pharmacotherapy, 48*(6), 741-751.

Zhang, Y., He, D., Sang, Y. (2013). Facebook as a platform for health information and communication: A case study of a diabetes group. *Journal of Medical Systems, 37*(3), 9942-9953. [http://dx.doi.org/10.1007/s10916-013-9942-7]

Zhang, Y., Sun, Y., Kim, Y. (2017). The influence of individual differences on consumer's selection of online sources for health information. *Computers in Human Behavior,* Elsevier Ltd. *67*, 303-312.

Zheng, Y. (2014). Patterns and motivations of young adults' health information acquisitions on Facebook. *Journal of Consumer Health on the Internet, 18*(2), 157-175. [http://dx.doi.org/10.1080/15398285.2014.902275]

Zickmund, S.L., Hess, R., Bryce, C.L., McTigue, K., Olshansky, E., Fitzgerald, K., Fischer, G.S. (2008). Interest in the use of computerized patient portals: role of the provider–patient relationship. *Journal of general internal medicine, 23*(1), 20-26.

SUBJECT INDEX

www.ingramcontent.com/pod-product-compliance
Lightning Source LLC
Chambersburg PA
CBHW041719210326
41598CB00007B/711